DEEP END of the POOL WORKOUTS

No-Impact Interval Training and Strength Exercises

Melisenda Edwards, MS
Katalin Wight, PT

Foreword by Shirley Archer, JD, MA

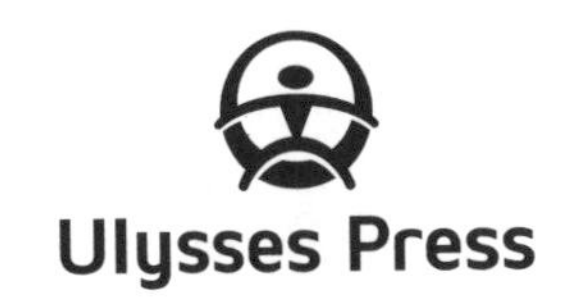

Ulysses Press

Published in the United States by
Ulysses Press
P.O. Box 3440
Berkeley, CA 94703
www.ulyssespress.com

ISBN: 978-1-61243-666-1
Library of Congress Control Number 2016957512

Printed in United States by United Graphics Inc.
10 9 8 7 6 5 4 3 2 1

Acquisitions: Bridget Thoreson
Managing Editor: Claire Chun
Editor: Lily Chou
Proofreader: Lauren Harrison
Indexer: Sayre van Young
Front cover and interior design: what!design @ whatweb.com
Photos: © Jesslyn Marie Braught and © Cassandra Powell except underwater shots © Dr. John Winnie Jr.
Interior illustrations: Jessica Lohmeier
Layout: Jake Flaherty
Models: Arianna Celis, Chris Edwards, Melisenda Edwards, Roger Fischer, Mitch Hanson, Trevon Hegel, Bridget Hoopes, Colter Mumford, Ross Snider

Distributed by Publishers Group West

This book is dedicated to our family, friends, and clients.

***

To my dad, for encouragement to follow my passion; Barb, the hardest client I've ever converted; and Kayleigh, the heart who connects two families and for making me appreciate every day of my life.

—Melis

To my family and my dearest friends, Melis and Joy:
Your love, support and encouragement create the solid foundation for all that I do. My heart overflows with love and gratitude for you.

—Katalin

Contents

Foreword

My first meeting with Melis Edwards was 20 some years ago when she came to my class as she was preparing for the Western States 100-mile endurance run. At the time, I was the director of a large group-fitness program at the Palo Alto Family YMCA in Palo Alto, California, that featured both aquatic and land-based classes.

After a few classes, I thought Melis would be an excellent fit as a deep water instructor, as deep water training perfectly complements the impact of many hours of outdoor trail-running. I knew that someone with her commitment and enthusiasm would be an inspiration to her students. I introduced her to another deep water running instructor on our staff, Sharon Svensson, DC, an Ironman (woman) athlete, and I referred her to another Silicon Valley–based facility, where I myself was also a deep water instructor. Melis quickly became one of the most popular teachers.

I've long been a passionate enthusiast of water fitness as well as other exercise modalities, and coauthored the book *YMCA Water Fitness for Health* (Human Kinetics, Inc., 2000), edited by leading international water fitness expert Mary E. Sanders, Ph.D., Fellow of the American College of Sports Medicine (FACSM), and adjunct professor in the School of Medicine at the University of Nevada, Reno. I authored *The Everything Weight Training Book* (Adams Media, 2002), which was the first strength-training book on the market to include a chapter on how to use the weight of water for muscle conditioning.

As a master trainer to fitness professionals, I traveled worldwide providing continuing education on the benefits of and skills required for effective aquatic training. I served as chair of the Water Fitness Committee for the IDEA Health & Fitness Association, worked with the Aquatic Exercise Association, the Aquatic Therapy and Rehabilitation Institute, the Arthritis Foundation Aquatic Program, and Hydrorider, creators of an innovative aquabike. I even served as a fitness model for Speedo aquatic fitness training gear ads! Through these experiences, I've had the privilege to meet top leaders in the field of hydro exercise and to be exposed to the breadth of training resources in aquatic fitness worldwide.

Here, in *Deep End of the Pool Workouts: No-Impact Interval Training and Strength Exercises,* Melis Edwards has created a valuable new addition to the body of knowledge that supports the tremendous benefits of hydro training. Melis has synthesized the many lessons from her 20-year career of teaching hydro exercise, coaching marathon and triathlon programs, personal training, and working with athletes and enthusiasts of all ages and levels of ability. She has created a comprehensive guide that's useful for both exercise enthusiasts and athletes as well as trainers and coaches.

Deep water training is significantly different from shallow water aquatic exercise. What I particularly love about *Deep End of the Pool Workouts: No-Impact Interval Training and Strength Exercises* is the emphasis on form and detailed explanations on why form matters. Without correct form, especially in the water, injury risks are increased. This is explained clearly with each exercise description, and modifications are provided to accommodate everybody at every level of proficiency. Another treasure in the book is the chapter dedicated to workout design. In this chapter, she provides 10 sample workouts with tips on how to organize them in an overall training plan.

This is a valuable book. It's an essential addition to the library of any coach or water fitness trainer. It provides access to information that every exercise enthusiast or elite athlete needs most—how to cross-train in the water for better performance and health. It's my privilege and honor to recommend it to you.

Shirley Archer, JD, MA
author of *Fitness 9 to 5: Easy Exercises for the Working Week*

Preface

I was first introduced to hydro running after spraining an ankle during track and field at De Anza College in Cupertino, California. At that time, I was on a team but I wasn't wholly committed to running; I spent more time figuring out ways to get out of it than actually train. I questioned anything my coaches asked me to do (in reflection, at that time I was an uncoachable athlete...but that's another story).

Because I didn't train properly, I often found myself injured. After a particular ankle injury, the coaches "threw me in the pool" to rehabilitate. I mean literally. The memory of being in my running clothes and shoes, treading water in the southeast corner of the De Anza high-dive pool, still stands out. I didn't understand how this could be helpful to my sprained ankle. It actually made me question my desire to run and compete. Suffice it to say, that experience turned me off of anything water-related for years. That was 1985.

Jump forward almost 10 years. This not-so-good 3-mile cross-country runner of the past, who used to go out too fast against her coach's advice and burn out within the first mile, had already completed a couple of marathons and worked her way through a 50k and a 50-miler. Strange as it sounds, I was also training for The Eagle, a 100-mile trail race in Canada.

Sometime during that 10 years I got serious about running. In the process of learning how to "endurance run," with assistance from my mentor and friend Kristina Irvin, D.C., I experienced all the glories of self-induced training problems: exhaustion issues, hypernatremia/hyponatremia, strains, sprains, and tendinitis. It was the hip tendinitis, so severe that I could barely lift my legs when walking, let alone trying to run, that drove me back to the pool.

I began taking a water aerobics class with Shirley Archer (author, speaker, and IDEA Fitness Instructor of the Year), an instructor at the Decathlon Club in Santa Clara. Since it seemed to be helping, Shirley suggested that I try water running with Sharon Svensson, DC, in Palo Alto. Sharon had been a pro-marathoner in the late '70s and early '80s, as well as an Ironman triathlete. Shirley felt that I could connect with her as an athlete, and I did. I started attending classes and learned that hydro running, when done right, didn't just heal my injured body but could also be used for training in lieu of running.

In 1995, under the direction of Shirley, I learned how to teach water fitness, and within a year I was instructing others in deep water interval training. I was first hired at the YMCA in Palo Alto and then took a position as a personal trainer and "hydro" instructor at the place where my career truly took off: the Decathlon Club (now called Bay Club Santa Clara). I began introducing hydro exercise to groups I was coaching at the "D-Club" and Courtside Club (CC) in Los Gatos as well. At CC, I used hydro exercise in a several-month half-marathon training program consisting of hydro mid-week and land runs on the weekends. Following this program, all of the participants either achieved their same times or produced personal bests. From both my personal experience as well as the successes my athletes experienced, I realized that hydro exercise was turning out to be an excellent training method that not only built aerobic ability but also produced power and speed.

Even with undeniable and rewarding success working with athletes, some of my favorite memories are of instructing seniors. I found that in many facilities, working with the aging population meant treating them with "kid gloves." However, I discovered that being a senior didn't always mean that their workouts needed to be easy. I found that this population could embrace and benefit from deep water interval training just as easily as athletes.

I noticed that when transitioning seniors to the deep end of the pool, they began remarking on how much better their bodies felt. Though the workouts were a bit tougher, they continued to express their satisfaction with "healthy" soreness and surprise with the development of muscles they didn't know they had. This population would regularly comment that they still had the rewards of shallow water workouts (i.e., decreased arthritic pain, increased flexibility) but now felt muscular strength and even more flexibility.

The transition of progressing water aerobic devotees to the deep end of the pool wasn't always easy; in some cases, participants left the class because they were drawn back to their familiar, "normal" workout. It was rough trying to convince these individuals to begin a new type of workout. What finally compelled the reluctant ones to come back were the participants who spoke up and constantly commented on how good they were feeling. My proudest moment was when I won over a former naysayer, Barb Trisler. What started out as a very tense departure from the pool on those initial "deep water" days has turned into a friendship that has lasted to today.

If you want a real workout that doesn't hurt your body but helps it, this is the exercise for you.

—Barbara, hydro exerciser for 30-plus years

Fast forward more than a few years: At age 45, I decided to expand my love and passion for health and wellness and chose to pursue a master's degree in health promotion. In doing so, I was able to broaden my career as a fitness instructor and coach, and further my role as an educator. My background as a credentialed teacher, through the understanding of class management and how to generate lesson plans, has always helped me in the fitness world. These skills naturally supported me in developing effective, progressive training programs.

Several years ago I began seriously batting around the idea to write a book on this type of exercise. "You should write a book, Melis" was something I heard from my trainees, friends, and associates. This notion steadily grew on me and the vision of a book took form. I began imagining a collaborative effort with friends and colleagues, and a platform to share my passion and my years of accumulated knowledge and experience.

I actually started working on two book ideas, one on running (since it's one of my passions) and the other on deep water fitness. This process included researching what was on the market. It was only then that I realized that there was definitely something missing in the area of water fitness—I couldn't find a comprehensive book on how to perform deep water interval training (which is also referred to as hydro interval training). I dropped the running book entirely and focused on deep water fitness. My continued research found many peer-reviewed articles in major scientific journals supporting my views on the benefits of hydro interval training, substantiating what I knew to be true. At the same time, I didn't want to do this project alone, so I convinced my friend of 30 years, Katalin Wight, to join me. Her insights into potential precautions from a physical therapist's point of view would serve to be valuable for anyone reading the book. The project then took on a life of its own, the book unfolding naturally into what you'll read in the coming pages.

Introduction

When thinking of working in water, you might visualize a group class with everyone facing one side of the pool, watching the instructor move through the choreographed workout. That's not the training you'll find in this book. Instead, imagine a track-style, interval-based, coached workout conducted in the deep end of a pool. The coach is on the pool deck looking into the water to watch the participants' motions as they travel in a loosely organized group through the deep end of the water. Each student performs the exercises at their own pace and intensity, depending on their individual needs. The coach verbally guides and modifies individuals' moves, demonstrating as needed, all while timing the intervals and calling out various intensities. This is hydro interval training (HIT), and it attracts athletes because they know real-time coaching brings proven results. Fitness enthusiasts have also easily embraced this workout style, which effectively improves their performance.

Hydro interval training utilizes clearly defined guidelines for form and technique to maximize benefits and minimize excessive stresses due to the higher forces required to move the body against water's resistance. The workouts incorporate speed, endurance, power, strength, and stretching; most exercises cover a greater range of motion than land-based workouts because of the participant's buoyancy. Done properly, these workouts can be very demanding. I've found that experienced athletes tend to progress and advance quickly and truly feel they're getting a valuable and effective training session. I've been told by an avid swimmer (a six-time Ironman athlete who I trained with HIT) that swimming 3,000 meters can be easier than one of my classes!

If you'd like to learn what professional athletes and fitness enthusiasts already know about deep water training, read on for extensive information on how to effectively navigate the waters in a group, design a workout program for your individual needs, and coach or instruct others in HIT.

PART 1

Before You Begin

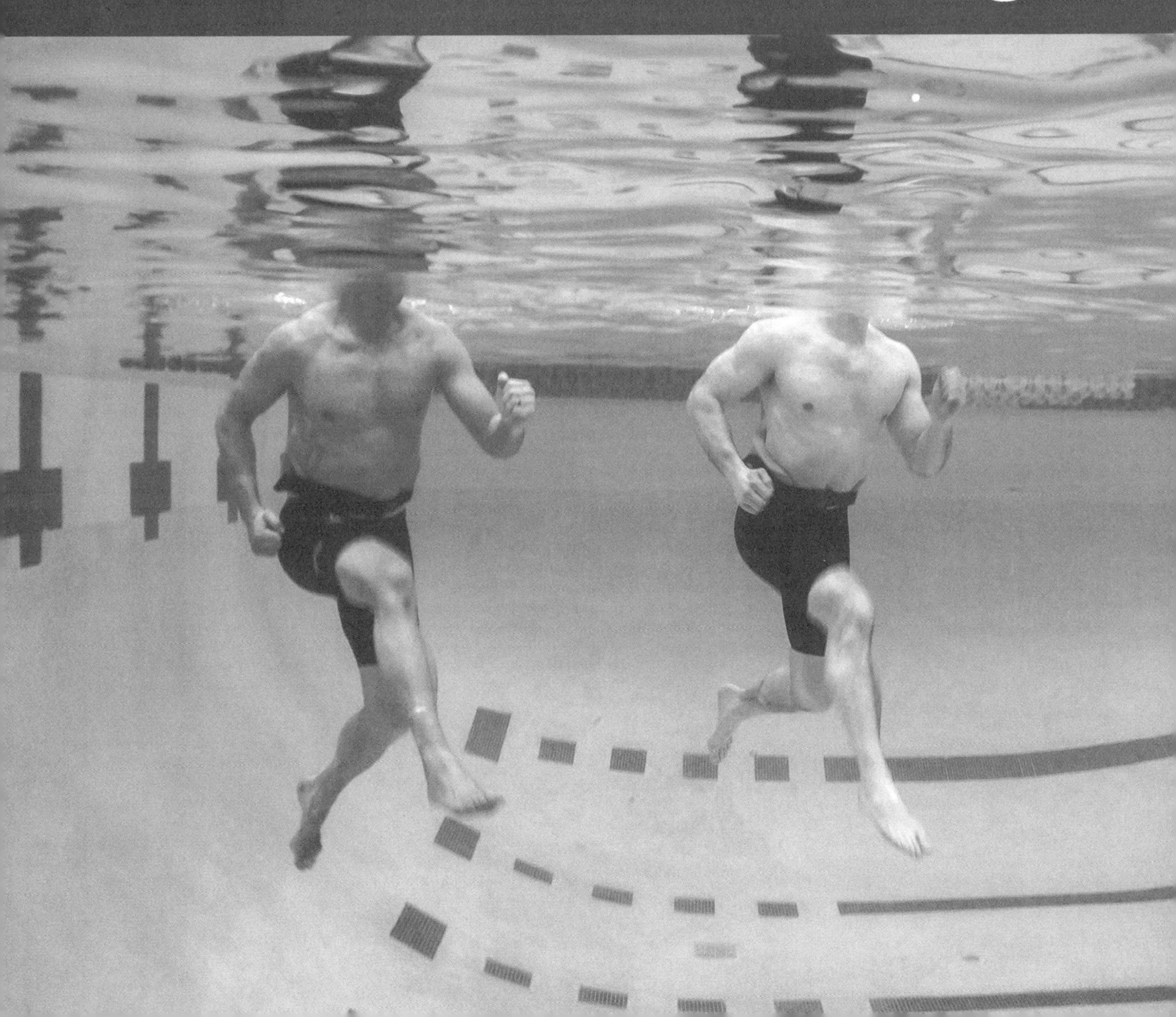

CHAPTER 1

Deep Water Training: What Am I Getting Into?

Deep water training is fitness training that happens in a pool without your feet touching the floor. You may be thinking, "Isn't that the definition of swimming?" Far from it. In hydro interval training (HIT), the type of deep water training found in this book, you'll be challenged with intense and demanding workouts that rival land-based training. This unique environment taxes strength and endurance in ways that are difficult to duplicate on land, with many benefits and advantages that are only recently being recognized. This fluid medium supports our weight and, because of its density, resists our movement in all directions, making it a near-perfect, no-impact, high-resistance exercise platform. My primary goal here is to shed light on the many benefits of training in water and to encourage curious, even skeptical, readers and fitness enthusiasts to take on a new, powerful, and unconventional approach to fitness.

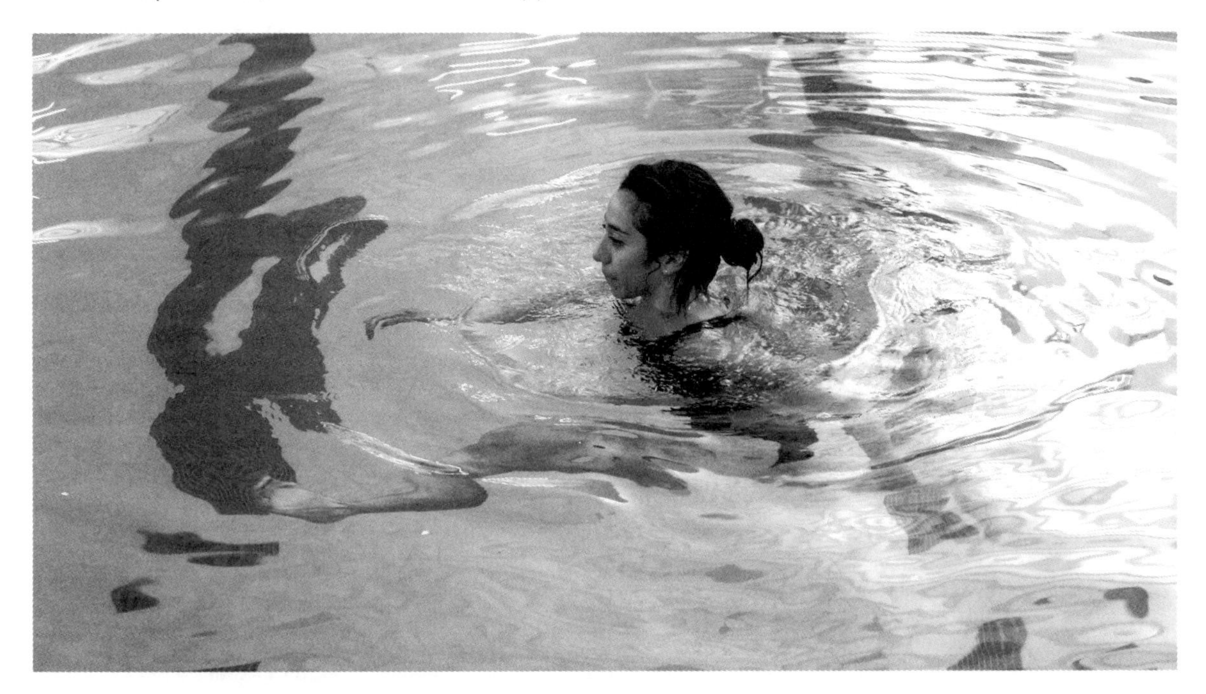

Whether you're a runner, cross trainer, triathlete, soccer player, or simply interested in increasing your overall fitness or athletic performance, wouldn't you want to use a method that's kinder to your joints while simultaneously maximizing gains? This platform is water, and this book will help your athletic performance no matter your sport.

I didn't anticipate the dramatic improvements in performance, endurance, and comfort level that I've realized since starting [the] program. These full-body, intense, low-impact workouts have made me a more well-rounded athlete.

—Bridget, naval engineer/scientist and amateur runner, dancer, cyclist, and sports enthusiast

Working in water is not a new concept. The term "water aerobics" is quite recognizable; community pool facilities typically offer these popular low-intensity, low-impact exercise classes. Lesser known is the more advanced water-based training, which is a powerful and effective tool currently used by many collegiate and professional athletes. My career has been spent gathering information and experiences on water training, attending numerous training courses, observing many coaches, and reading countless articles and books. I've helped hockey players, triathletes, runners, mountain bikers, and fitness enthusiasts use water as part of their training to improve their performance and fitness. Based on these experiences, I've adapted water training into the exercise method presented in this book.

As an athlete who has personally used this book's exact program very successfully for over 20 years, I've experienced all the concepts, techniques, and rewards of deep water training. In addition, I've trained many top-notch athletes using these workouts, helping them to maintain and even improve fitness while recovering from injury, as well as used HIT as a part of an overall training plan to increase athletic performance. While there have been many books written about water aerobics, only a few promoted the deep end of the pool. This book combines my passion, experience, research, and knowledge into a unique style of deep water training that I'm now sharing with you.

A STEP BACK IN TIME AND A LEAP FORWARD

The history of using water for healing goes as far back as 863 B.C. to Bath, England, where it's said the city's founder was supposedly cured of leprosy after bathing in the area's hot springs. However, water in the form of hot springs was mostly used for soaking ailing bodies, and was prescribed for everything from gout to dry skin to arthritis.[1] Water's transition from medicine to therapy to a training tool came sometime in the early to mid-20th century. Early uses included treating paralyzed patients in wooden tanks and utilizing hot springs as pools for physical therapy.[2] In *Technique of Underwater Gymnastics: A Study in Practical Application* (1937), possibly the first book written on water training, Dr. Charles Leroy Lowman detailed aquatic rehabilitation and the theory behind deep water training, from program design to specifics on the use of heated salt pools to decrease bacteria growth. In his book he stated, "The chief advantage of water as a medium for bodily exercise is that the entire body, or any of its parts, can move in any plane. From the standpoint of technique, the most important use of this advantage lies in its allowance of all sorts of trunk movements which cannot be executed similarly elsewhere."[3]

Supported by more documented research and publications, the last 20 years have seen a significant rise in use and popularity of water training. In 1997, Steve Tarpinian and Dr. Brian Awbrey wrote a book called *Water Workouts* featuring many well-known athletes of the 1980s and 1990s—Bo Jackson, George Brett, Joan Benoit-Samuelson, Carl Lewis, and Nancy Kerrigan, all of whom used the deep water of a pool to rehabilitate their injuries and rebound to a competitive level in their respective sports. Tarpinian and Awbrey also noted that when track and field great Carl Lewis won nine Olympic gold medals at his peak in the '80s, he didn't just use water training for injury rehabilitation—he also used water running for his "spring" and "balance" work.[4]

So why would a world-class athlete step into the pool instead of going out and training on the track? One reason is recovery. One, if not the biggest, training limiter is the amount of time it takes to recover from a workout, especially from the routine damage done to bodies by impact with the ground or by the strain of heavy-weight training sessions, for example. Performing an intense session in the water environment alone doesn't seem to produce the same levels of muscle soreness and damage as is experienced following similar land-based exercise. As an article in the *Journal of Strength and Conditioning Research* noted, "the water environment influenced the absence of significant muscle damage. This type of exercise protocol may be appropriate for situations in which limited muscle tissue damage is desired."[5]

In a recent *Sports Health* article on examining plyometric training in the pool, research revealed that water reduced impact of "up to 62% in peak impact forces…compared with their land-based equivalents."[6] Carl Lewis was clearly on to something; he had found a way to increase his training volume and intensity without subjecting his body to impact injury, thus reducing his need for longer recovery periods. More recently, Maria Hutsick, athletic director of the 2002 USA women's Olympic ice hockey team and former director of sports medicine at Boston University, used deep water training to train her Olympic athletes longer and harder, more days each week, with less trauma and injury to muscles and joints. Her women's hockey team won an Olympic silver medal in 2002. Currently, Abby Rugy, a coach for Carmichael Training Systems, prescribes deep water training to triathletes during the off season, reducing accumulated stress and enhancing recovery from the long racing season, while helping to maintain the high levels of fitness gained from competing.

WHY TRAIN IN DEEP WATER?

You might think starting off in the shallow end would be a better strategy than plunging into the deep side, which may be seen as more difficult. I disagree—I find that the work in deep water produces increased body awareness more quickly because of the constant requirement for core stability, defined body positions, and limb movements. As a result, when an individual migrates to shallow water, the newly enhanced dynamic body awareness and control helps maintain stability, coordination, and training intensities.

Promoting deep water training doesn't exclude shallow water work—quite the contrary. A 2010 *International Journal of Aquatic Research and Education* article found that "aquatic-based plyometrics have the potential to decrease impact forces as compared with land-based plyometric training. The decrease in distributed impact force is largely due to the properties of water in relation to fluid density and buoyancy."[7] Consider the plyometric single-foot hop, which cannot be performed in deep water. This maneuver is beneficial to land sports and is used to increase power, specifically for the acceleration and propulsion phase, which is generated primarily by the lower leg muscles. This hop can be used in training for any sport that involves a "pushing off" motion (running, sprinting) or jumping action (basketball, figure skating).

I started deep water training when I developed some serious joint injuries and tendinitis from all the tennis and soccer I was doing. It became a wonderful alternative to the high-impact training I performed daily by providing intense resistance training with little impact on the joints. I met some other pretty amazing athletes with and without injuries, and folks of various ages and fitness levels looking for a fun group environment and challenging workouts. I loved being able to achieve full range of body motion, which promoted deep stretching in our exercises while simultaneously being able to target specific muscle groups. I always feel amazing after a deep water running workout.

—Wu, avid cross-country mountain biker and chemical engineer

With the forces of gravity at play, a plyometric hop on land is a strenuous exercise to perform, especially when injured. When done in the shallow end of the pool, the impact through the leg is significantly reduced.[8] If recovering from an ankle injury for example, choosing to train with this exercise in shallow water would allow the initiation of a dynamic exercise earlier than on land.

Furthermore, deep water training could be initiated almost immediately to maintain full-body fitness and range of motion of the ankle.

BENEFITS OF SUSPENSION

A suspended state truly challenges a person's coordination and balance, forcing increased muscle engagement with every motion in order to stabilize the body in the correct upright position. By purposefully changing body positions, speeds, and interval durations, you can get the workout you want from light, moderate, or intense exercise to aerobic training to even bouts of anaerobic training. So besides water, the most important tool in HIT is a flotation belt, which allows you to concentrate on doing a wide range of exercises correctly and at varying intensities without having to worry too much about keeping your head above water. For the seasoned athlete, the belt allows for keen focus on form to target muscle recruitment, and promotes significant full-body strength gains that carry over to all other activities.

Being suspended in deep water changes the kinetic chain, making the motions open (ungrounded) rather than closed (grounded). A closed kinetic chain movement is when that part of your body is in contact with a stabilizing solid surface (for example, the ground or pool bottom). Closed chains are the norm for the legs in land-based fitness or shallow water aerobics. When the kinetic chain is open, especially for all four limbs, the instability created requires much more core engagement to gain a solid foundation in order to perform a move. This is amplified in deep water training because ungrounded movements are intensified by the drag encountered in the water. Core stability is fundamental for HIT, which is why I focus on it throughout the book.

If you're relatively injury free and running many miles a week, you should ask yourself, "How much longer can this last?" Studies looking at runners' long-term durability are not encouraging. Roughly 65% of runners experience either chronic minor injuries or periodic injuries serious enough that they need to stop running.[9] Impacts on your body add up over time. Consider that during every run you take, the strike force of your foot hitting the ground can be up to six times your own body weight depending on speed, style, and running ability.[10] This means that a 150-pound runner could experience 600 to 900 pounds of impact force with each foot strike. Furthermore, when running, each foot strikes the ground up to 2,000 times per mile—a tremendous number of high-force impacts on feet, knees, hips, and the lower back.[11] It's no wonder that two-thirds of us are running injured! Running on land isn't a bad thing. I love running—I'm an ultra distance runner and a seven-time Ironman finisher. I've run *thousands* of miles. What I believe, though, is that deep water training can help you extend your running, or any sport with high joint impact, for many more years to come.

Fast After 50: How to Race Strong for the Rest of Your Life by Joel Friel, one of the most eminent coaches of our time, looks at ways for athletes to maintain and even increase athletic performance as they age.[12] He observes that endurance athletes gradually change to longer, slower distances, foregoing high-intensity training to spare joints and allow for easier recovery as they age. Because of this approach to training, he believes athletic performance dwindles. To counter this decline, Friel advocates that athletes continue high-intensity interval work, even into their 70s. I build on that concept and suggest that some of this high-intensity interval work can be done in the water, sparing aging joints from impacts and minimizing recovery time.

Just think about using deep water training for your own workouts—less impact on joints and less soreness, but with the intensity you want. The water setting allows a higher level of intensity, yields great results, and is more conducive to preservation of the health of the active and aging body than a 100% land-based fitness program. Remember the 2002 USA women's Olympic ice hockey team? How about nine-time Olympic medalist Carl Lewis, who used water training regularly? He trained unconventionally in order to continue competing at a very high level. His career spanned four Olympic Games (16 years) and I believe that some of that success in part can be attributed to training in the water.

LET HIT BE YOUR NEXT STEP

Water training is an activity coaches have been using for years to improve their athletes' performance and help with injury recovery, yet there are few guides available for understanding the detailed methods behind working in deep water. This book provides teaching tips, cues and terms to use, health and safety advice, and extensive advice for coaching HIT from the deck. Sample workouts illustrate how to use specific exercises to customize your workouts. Use this book alone or in conjunction with other training guides such as the Aquatic Exercise Association's *Aquatic Fitness Professional Manual*, especially if your intention is to become a trainer or coach. It's important for readers to understand that training in the water can be adapted for people of most ages and abilities, from fitness newbies to professional athletes. Keeping participants engaged for the long run is one of our primary goals.

Consider the setbacks you've experienced when you couldn't train in your primary sport. Do you remember how much cardiovascular conditioning and muscle strength you lost when you were "out" for a week, a month, or longer? If you're 20 to 40 years old, recognize that your body will age; what can you do now to keep you strong and fit until your 70s? How about those of us that are in our 50s, 60s 70s...90s? Our minds and hearts still want to race, perform, and excel, yet can our bodies take the continuous stresses and strains? How do we pull this together to still be successful, active, and thriving?

Deep water training can answer all these questions for you.

CHAPTER 2

Getting Ready for HIT

Exercises performed in the aquatic environment have different physiological and biomechanical responses from those carried out on dry land due to the influence exerted by the physical properties of water on the human body.

—from the *Journal of Human Kinetics*[13]

As a coach and personal trainer, I'm disheartened when other coaches or trainers of various sports are resistant to working their athletes in the water. Typically this has been due to the lack of knowledge of how water training can boost performance or the belief that water training means the athlete must be injured. I know personally that the benefits of deep water interval workouts can carry over to land training and sports. Running in general causes repetitive impact on joints, especially the knee. In ultrarunning (distances greater than the traditional 26.2-mile marathon), the effect is amplified by the volume of running necessary to prepare for the longer races. I knew my joints couldn't handle that volume on land alone. So in 2015, while training for a 50k race, I supplemented my regimen with 1- to 2-hour sessions of pool running twice a week. Water training allowed me to increase my mileage each week without suffering additional ground-force trauma in my knees. And demonstrating the fallacy about water training, almost every time I was exercising in the pool, others asked if I was injured. When I said I wasn't, they often asked whether what I was doing really "worked."

One of the greatest advantages of working in the water is that there's very little, if any, muscle pain or soreness the following day after performing an intense deep water workout. It doesn't matter how hard the workout was—there isn't the same muscle pain that would be felt after a hard track workout, for example.[14] In a nutshell: No ground-force impacts results in the muscles being worked without the pounding effect of the legs meeting the ground.

In 2011, with the help of Melis, I began training for not only my first Ironman but my first triathlon, my first marathon, and my first introduction into road biking. The first few months of training went by without a hitch. I then made an amateur mistake of buying a new pair of running shoes and switching overnight from running in zero-drop shoes to fully supported, padded cross-trainers. I went for a 13-mile trail run followed by sitting in a three-hour study session. The next morning, I couldn't take one step without limping and wincing from the pain in my hip flexor.

I immediately saw a physical therapist. To my horror, he informed me that if I wanted any chance of even starting the race, I'd have to withhold from running for at least two months! I walked out of my appointment in tears. When Melis heard the tale, she patiently consoled me, asked me if I trusted her, and told me that I'd just have to start water running with her multiple days a week.

My initial reaction was drenched in skepticism. But I had no other choice. For the next two to three months, I converted my run sets to water running sets and drills that Melis prescribed. My hip slowly healed and less than three months until race day, I was told that I could attempt a very short, outdoor run. It was within my first two runs on land that I discovered my skepticism about water running couldn't have been more wrong! My first run was a 6-miler and, although I tried to take it easy, I discovered that my speed was no slower than it had been three months prior. My second land run was a 12-mile "training run," and it wasn't until I finished and looked at my time that I realized that I had PR'd—I unintentionally made a personal record during a 12-mile training run, after not running on land in three months! I was astonished.

I continued supplementing my run sets with water running until about a month before race day. I went on to complete my very first Ironman, coming in fourth in my age group and in the top 10th percentile for women overall. I would've never made it to the start of that race, let alone the end, without Melis's support. I'm now walking proof that water running is not only a legitimate alternative to land running but could possibly even be the way to go.

—Kelcie, Ironman finisher and water resource engineer

COMMITTING TO HIT: PRESUMPTION VERSUS REALITY

Everyone has a history with fitness and a personal motivation behind their commitment to exercise. Maybe it's to get in better shape, lose weight, decrease stress, or master a sport. Whatever your ultimate goal, I want HIT to become part of these stories.

The 2016 exercise guidelines by American College of Sports Medicine as well as the World Health Organization have suggested that adults participate in 150 minutes (or 2.5 hours weekly) of moderate intensity exercise every week.[15] This training should incorporate flexibility, resistance, and neuromuscular training—everything hydro interval training incorporates in one workout method. Unfortunately, the truth is that many adults are not meeting this minimum amount. If you fall into this category, deep water training might be the exercise that will draw you into the world of fitness.

> **I was introduced to deep water interval training as an aspiring cyclist for both road and mountain biking. The first thing I noticed were my sore hamstrings. I found that the resistance in deep water was great for my hamstrings and also a great training regimen for cycling during the winter months when getting out in the ice/snow wasn't practical. Two additional benefits came with the deep water interval training. The first was the ability to stretch my hamstrings on every stroke. The second was getting a good core workout, which didn't happen during regular spinning classes. I found that deep water interval training was as hard (or even harder) than a high-intensity spin class.**
>
> —Ross, engineering professor and cyclist

What I really love about HIT is that no matter your athletic ability or experience, you *will* work, and you *will* work hard. A beginner participant and accomplished athlete both burn calories the same or even faster than on land because so many muscles are being used simultaneously in the deep water. There have been numerous research studies looking into the calories burned when performing deep water interval training; it's generally upward of 600 to 700 calories per hour, or approximately 11.5 calories per minute.[16] The low end of the scale starts around 300 calories (equivalent to a strong 3-mile-per-hour walk pace) on up to the above-mentioned higher ends.[17] In this respect, deep water training is comparable to land training; it all depends upon the intensity.

If you exercise regularly or are a high-caliber athlete, this book could be the next best step you take in your training. For some individuals, especially those who put in high mileage, performing land-based exercises five or more times per week can be too taxing on their joints. Personally, as a long-time distance runner, I've never been able to run every day, even when training for 100-mile ultra races. When I tried running daily, it didn't take long for my knees and hips to start screaming at me. Using deep water to supplement my land-based training was the key to unlocking my ability to participate in a sport like ultrarunning.

Another excellent benefit of deep water training is that it improves your posture when on land. Many of the strokes you'll learn incorporate significant core engagement, with an emphasis placed on strengthening the muscles on the back side of the body, from the hamstrings and glutes up to the mid- and upper-back, while stabilizing with the abdominals. This approach combats the all-too-common turtle posture, where the neck and shoulder are hunched with the pelvis tilted backward.

DEEP WATER TRAINING ISN'T FOR EVERYONE

I've personally worked with many individuals in the deep water after consultation with their physical therapist and/or doctors. Individuals who suffered from conditions such as plantar fasciitis, shin splints, ACL surgery, runner's knee, iliotibial (IT) band syndrome, Achilles tendinitis, back strains to herniations, hip replacement surgery, and more have successfully participated in hydro interval training.

However, I've also found individuals who simply shouldn't jump into the deep end first. Even though movements take place in the seemingly supportive water environment, pushing too hard in any medium while rehabilitating can result in setbacks. The pool is different from other fitness settings, so it's important to consider not just the activities being performed but the overall health and condition of a prospective participant.

Whether a facilitator or a participant, it's crucial to follow the guidelines of a medical professional when starting any exercise program. The advice is simple: If you've had any recent or past injury/surgery, consult with your physician or physical therapist. This includes individuals with high blood pressure, cardiac problems, and emphysema or other respiratory issues.

It may sound overly cautious but experience has shown me that deep water training isn't appropriate for some people. An example: Only last year a person new to water fitness attended an interval-based workout I was instructing, but she failed to mention that she had a Cesarean section only two months prior. Her doctor told her it was okay to get in the water for water aerobics, so she came to my class. She didn't mention this *major* detail to me until I literally saw her looking green with nausea. The intensity of a HIT workout and the involvement of the abdominal muscles is definitely not recommended so soon after a Cesarean.

Deep End of the Pool Workouts isn't a rehabilitation book that gently works your muscles. If this is what you're seeking, this is not the book for you.

TRAIN SMART: MAKE HIT WORKOUTS WORK FOR YOU

Using water allows you to train as you want since "a wide repertoire of movement is possible, allowing proprioception, body balance, strength, and aerobic exercises."[18] The resistance you encounter when moving in the water can make your workout any effort you desire.

In fact, the harder or faster you push against the water, the harder the workout becomes. Water training can be like land training—do an easy workout one day or a hard interval the next. Within each workout, you can increase or decrease the intensity to what you're seeking, depending on the day and your training regime. Also, training in deep water isn't something that will progressively get less intense over time, as some would think. Water training is a combination of cardiovascular conditioning, strength training, and stretching. It doesn't have to be one intensity. As you master the strokes, strength and coordination improve, giving you even more opportunity to challenge your body, in some cases learning to use muscles in ways that are improbable on land.

The simultaneous open kinetic chain movements of the limbs during hydro interval training require additional muscles that aren't used as readily when on land. For example, when runners or cyclists return to land, they're stronger and can engage their core for a stronger performance. Of course, not every water workout MUST be an interval workout. Some of the best recovery workouts I've had are in the water. The supportive environment allows the hips and limbs to stretch out, such as when performing the Cross-Country stroke. Remember, you can control the effort; you control the fitness focus.

It's important to note that there's a learning curve to HIT. New athletes trying interval training in the water for the first time may feel that the workout is too easy. This is because they haven't learned to work within the water as well as someone with experience. Deep water interval training involves the challenging combination of learning coordinated movements while developing full-body strength. This would be similar to a land-based boot camp or indoor cycling class—no one leaves thinking the workout was easy. Be patient and keep in mind that, just like with any new activity, there will be a period of discovery and assimilation. No matter one's body awareness, abilities, and physical prowess, I've rarely put someone in the pool that was able to perfectly perform every stroke the first time. Plan on working in water at least a half-dozen times before you start to feel that you're mastering the stroke technique and form and manipulating the water to its full advantage.

Outside of this learning curve, some people may also experience difficulty breathing when submerged in water up to their necks. Water pressure on the body, limbs, and chest region can initially make it hard to take in a full breath of air. It's not always noticeable but, for some, it can leave them panting on the edge of the pool until their intercostal (muscles between the ribs) and other respiratory muscles become stronger. Strengthening of the muscles responsible for breathing is an additional benefit everyone will experience. When runners work in the water for several weeks they can actually experience an easier time breathing during land training.[19] This sensation is unique to water training. Even swimmers can achieve some of the added benefits of deep water training as they're typically not vertical in the water, but rather horizontal with lungs closer to the surface of the water. In the pool, the more submerged the body is, the more water pressure plays a role.

Yet, because of the intensities that can be achieved in water, it's important to use this training platform in the same manner as you would with training on land. With this in mind, I wouldn't put a person who's generally new to fitness through one of the advanced workouts in Chapter 6 without assessing their response to a more basic workout. Without being informed of exercise guidelines or potential responses,[20] new participants to water could go through the workout regardless of their form, but may work harder than intended due to their deconditioned state. It's important to provide proper guidance on efforts.

People fatigue quickly in water for the same reasons they do on land: being deconditioned, pushing too hard before they're ready, or not being recovered sufficiently from a prior workout or illness. It's important to recognize these situations and look for signs of exhaustion even in experienced athletes. Treat these individuals as you would in any other workout with longer recoveries and possibly less intensity until they recover and/or develop strength and stamina.

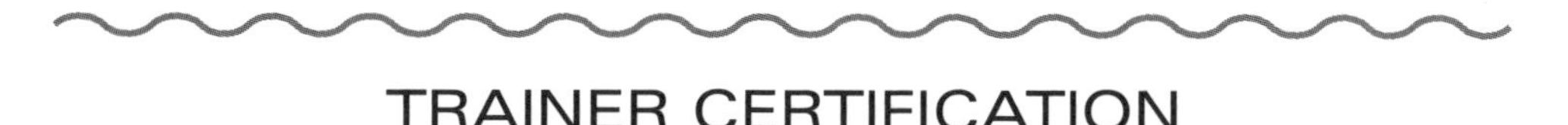

TRAINER CERTIFICATION

If your goal is to become a facilitator or trainer, being certified in ACSM, AEA, NASM, ACE, or another similar certifying program is recommended as you'll need to put your anatomy and physiology knowledge to use. You may find the PT Points (tips from a physical therapy perspective; see page 32) a helpful starting point on how to advise your clients on when they should consider entering the pool. For those who are using this book for personal use, the PT Points are written so that all readers can process the information, regardless of their training experience or education.

TOOLS OF THE TRADE

The wonderful thing about deep water training is that you don't need much equipment to start—just water deep enough to be suspended and a flotation belt or vest. I've worked in public pools, a private home pool in Belize, and in the oceans in Mexico, Kona, Maui, and Kauai—all with the same results. The only difference was the water: chlorine, bromine (saltwater pool), or sea. A bonus of being in the ocean is that you may not need a flotation device due to increased density and hydrostatic pressure. (Items float better in denser water and salt makes water denser.)

A flotation device isn't used to "cheat" or make a workout easier. It's primarily to keep the body in the most optimum position to perform the movements in the deep end. Without flotation, the participant's form typically falls apart. This can be seen in two ways with even the most basic moves, such as the Water Run (page 38). The first is where the pelvis moves back and the hips become hitched (see image at right), rather than staying in alignment with the shoulders as the legs kick forward. Another issue can be that a participant may lie back in the water, appearing almost to be on a recumbent bike in the water! This isn't to say that deep water training can't be performed without a belt, but I strongly recommend that all participants start with a flotation belt to optimize success. If it's not being used, additional attention must be paid to maintaining form.

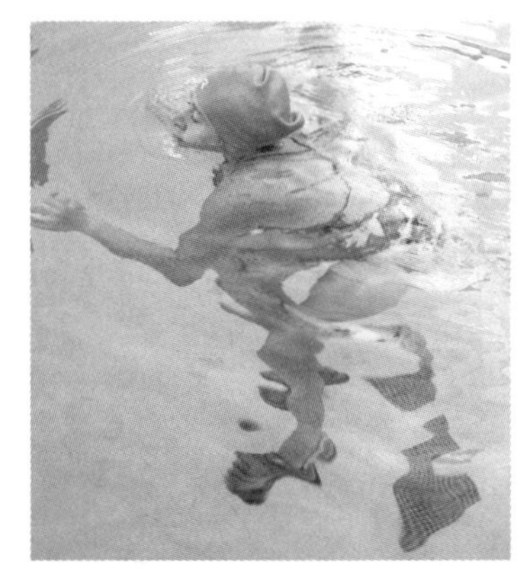

Water Run without a belt may contribute to incorrect form, seen as hitched hips.

The flotation belt provides the ability to control the overall heart rate, especially with intense workouts. Some deep water runners will forego the flotation belt in order to add another level of difficulty to the exercises, but this usually compromises proper form. Rather than simply doing the exercises as they were designed, beltless athletes wind up having to add awkward, peripheral movements to the exercise to keep themselves afloat. A beltless workout demands an enormous amount of extra energy just to keep the head above water, not to mention trying to perform the stroke correctly. Attempting to perform a majority of the workout sets in this book without a belt would have participants' heart rates hitting or exceeding threshold levels (85% or above). This was exactly the situation of my first experience over 30 years ago when I was thrown in the pool to train without a belt. It was so unpleasant that it kept me from water training for years. By using a flotation belt you can do the exercises correctly and at very high intensity, and if you feel you aren't getting enough of a workout with the flotation belt on, well, you simply aren't pushing hard enough.

Over the years I've used a variety of flotation devices, from belts, vests, dumbbells, and even cuffs that go on the wrists and/or ankles. I could write a separate chapter dedicated to the pros and cons of each. For this book, however, the only equipment mentioned for participants will be a standard flotation belt.

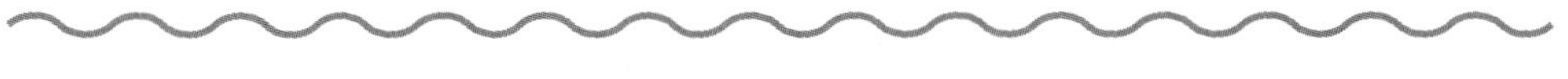

SHOWERING FOR THE POOL

No matter whether you're using a pool treated with chlorine or bromine, both can irritate your skin. One of the best habits to adopt is showering before and after using the pool. It's better for your skin and removes body oils, perspiration, cosmetics, and other body residues. When you don't shower, those clingy body substances get in the pool or stay on your skin and combine with chlorine, producing the strong chlorine smell. This strong smell is not a sign of a clean pool; it's actually a sign of a dirty pool. Typically, a healthy, managed pool has no strong smell! So please shower; it will help your skin *and* the pool.

Belt fit is important and is based on several factors, such as the type of belt and the buoyancy provided. You may need to experiment to some degree before finding the right one for your body and needs. Each can be worn on the front or the back; it's a matter of comfort and countering the flotation of the belt with your own "personal" flotation. If you have large breasts or a large abdomen, you may want to "counter" your buoyancy with the flotation belt to keep your body in an upright position. The belt should allow for your head to be above water when moving at a light aerobic effort. If your head sinks under water past your mouth, additional flotation is necessary. For example, an athlete who has several hundred pounds of lean body mass may need more flotation. In the early 2000s I worked with a muscular San Jose Sharks hockey player who sunk past his chin with just one belt around his abdomen. So I placed a second belt around his hips to solve the problem.

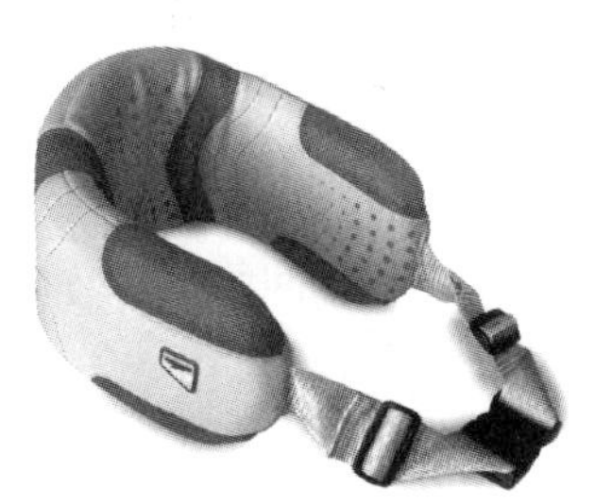

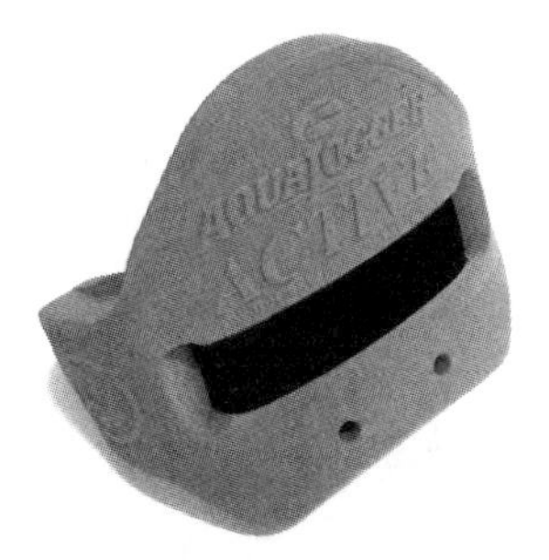

Different brands of flotation devices

Regardless of personal preference and fit requirements, the cost range is generally from $20 to $40 dollars. Many public pools provide this piece of equipment so you may not have to purchase one. This will allow you to experience various flotation belts to find the right one for you.

A note about pool noodles: It's difficult to do HIT using them. No matter where the noodle is located or held, it will inhibit proper movement of the limbs or cause unnecessary chaffing, especially if it were held around the back and under the armpit area or positioned between the legs.

Other Equipment. When I suggest deep water training to new people who are primarily land-based athletes, sometimes the first comment is that they don't have a swim suit. A regular swim suit works well but I let them know that a pair of shorts and a sports bra (for women) also works fine for this type of training. Companies are now incorporating more options for workout clothing that can be used for deep water training.

You can also throw on a pair of water shoes, no socks necessary. There are hydro-specific shoes on the market (Ryka, Avia, Sprint Aqua) that provide free movement of water through the shoes, which drain and dry out once you're out of the water. The shoes will create a bit more drag when the legs drive through the water with better engagement of the hamstrings. This isn't to say that the rest of the leg muscles aren't working! However, this additional drag can be too much strain for people who may be recovering from a hamstring injury.

Hydration during water exercise is as important as on land, so everyone should bring a water bottle. Time and time again, I'll see athletes show up to water training without water to drink.

Whether it's the mistaken belief that you won't get thirsty or the avoidance of needing to use a bathroom, I tell my clients to come with water and, if they need to take a bathroom break, get out of the water and take one.

Finally, there are some other items that I believe are necessary, specifically when training outside: sunscreen, sun shirts, caps, and sunglasses. My athletes (and myself) have been teased when getting into the pool with these items, but the sun is very bright, especially when reflected off the pool surface onto a face only inches away. Comfort and safety are always fundamental.

GENERAL CONSIDERATIONS

As with all exercise programs, if you're under the care of a physical or occupational therapist for a physical condition, injury, or fracture, or are recovering from a surgical procedure, it's vital that you consult with your therapist regarding this type of exercise, including the specific strokes and movements found in HIT. Your physical therapist will be the most qualified to provide you specific activity precautions and instructions. If you're solely under the care of a physician for any of the conditions mentioned, consult with them before engaging in deep water training.

While the exercises presented are not intended to be "rehabilitation," they certainly can be used to regain function and fitness and build levels of strength and stamina.

HEALTH ISSUES

If you have any chronic heart or lung conditions, gradually ease into any water exercises and pay careful attention to your body's responses and sensations. Immersion to the neck level has a significant effect on the heart and on circulation not experienced on land. The water pressure causes the heart to fill with more blood before each contraction, which means the heart must work harder to pump out the blood. Yet being immersed in water actually has the effect of decreasing heart rate in average pool temperatures, and can decrease blood pressure as well.[21] If you're not accustomed to water's unique influences on heart function, or if you have cardiac issues, consult your physician before starting deep water training. Serious heart conditions include but are not limited to:

- valvular insufficiency
- heart failure
- recent myocardial infarction/heart attack

Immersion in water also distinctly affects breathing and lung function. Water pressure compresses the chest area (and the entire body), which increases the effort needed to fill the lungs with air. This provides an opportunity for healthier individuals to strengthen the muscles used for breathing.[22] However, chronic lung conditions/diseases and congestive heart failure will likely affect your breathing abilities and comfort in the water. That being said, there are known benefits to exercising in water, such as:

- decreased edema/swelling and pain related to varicose veins
- increased blood flow
- decreased general body pains and stiffness
- decreased weight-bearing stress on the joints, including the spine
- improved balance and coordination on land that can reduce the risk of falling

ACTIVITY PRECAUTIONS

For those who struggle with chronic back issues and/or pain, your physical therapist can provide you guidance and/or training in how to strengthen the muscles of the spine or any of the other muscle groups to prepare you for HIT. While HIT provides an excellent means of achieving improved physical fitness and conditioning, be patient and proceed in a gradual fashion. Pay attention to how your body responds to and feels with the different strokes and movements. This experimentation will help determine the exercises or variations that best address your needs and objectives, accommodate your limitations, and keep you participating in the exercise regularly. Make adjustments as needed while still safely challenging yourself to get stronger. Being attentive and self-aware of your body is a valuable and empowering experience.

HIT is a full-body workout with all of the exercises performed in deep water without a fixed surface to stabilize the body. This alone causes a very different type of action and stressor on the joints than any land-based activity in which the ground provides stabilization. All the movements require heavy use of the abdominal and back/spinal muscle groups, from the neck down to the lower spine, any time the limbs are in motion. Core strength and stability not only allow for proper form, but protect the spine from exceeding its limits of stability and integrity.

The dynamic and powerful motions of the arms and legs rely heavily on the shoulder and hip joints. These joints are continuously under some degree of stress when moving the limbs against resistance. When it comes to strengthening and conditioning, this is one of the greatest benefits of working in water but can be a challenge when recovering from surgery or injury or when managing a chronic issue. In addition, changing arm or leg directions in water requires greater energy and strength than on land. The potential effects of this type of strenuous activity must be considered if you have conditions that involve any section of your spine/trunk/ribs, at any level, including but not limited to:

- muscular strain/trauma
- joint sprain
- fractures
- spinal (from the neck to the sacral/lower spine) and abdominal/intestinal surgery
- hernia/hernia repair
- abdominal muscle injuries
- internal infection/abscess
- C-section
- breast surgery or augmentation
- open-heart surgery

If you've had knee surgery, especially procedures that involve the cruciate ligaments, meniscus, or patella, you must consult your physical therapist or physician. The open-chain configuration of all the lower-limb exercises can stress the knee joint, which may not be advised.

Excessively tensing your shoulders into a shrug may cause neck/shoulder tension or pain. This can occur in strokes such as the Run if you prioritize power before proper form.

If you identify a significant imbalance in strength and power for any reason, pay special attention to related form issues found in the specific PT Points of each position or stroke and study the associated corrections in the Form Issues. This will promote development of more balanced movements and forces that will lead to maximal training benefits and support your fitness education.

Other factors to consider are exercise variables that require increased joint stability and muscle strength, such as:

- faster limb movement speeds
- further extension of the elbow and knee joints (no lockouts!)
- longer distances of the limbs away from the body

When combining these conditions, you further intensify the exercise. If you're experiencing discomfort or pain, reduce one or all of these factors.

As with any sort of physical activity, onset of pain is generally a sign that the body is being stressed in some way beyond the capacity of its strength, stability, and capability. If you experience pain during any of these activities, immediately adjust or modify the exercise by either changing body position, reducing power, slowing the movement, or reducing the duration. In some cases, the entire exercise should be replaced with a less intense variation or a different stroke altogether. If you're a trained athlete, continue to use your familiar methods of communication with your body, but be aware that, if you're new to deep water exercise, you may experience unfamiliar sensations and responses.

Considering the safety of coaches, trainers, and instructors, all demonstrations should be done with one foot planted on the pool deck. This position requires good balance so, if additional support is needed for your safety, plan ahead by using a chair, pool rail, or other equipment for balance assistance. Unless indicated differently, keep this in mind when reading about and learning the strokes.

Be safe and enjoy!

CHAPTER 3

Anatomy of Deep Water Exercise—You Aren't Just Floating

> *[Deep water fitness] is significantly underused and mostly misunderstood.... If executed correctly, however, water running will not only maintain performance but it will often even improve performance."*
>
> —Michael Moon, author of *Deep Water Exercise for High Performance Sport*[23]

Yes, you're actually floating...but it's nothing like the floating you may be picturing. There's no inner tube or raft with a drink holder. The reason most people tend to be turned off or uninspired by training in the water is that they don't understand how they'd benefit from adding it to their fitness program. They may associate water with play or being at the beach, or recall memories of watching a low-intensity water aerobics class. Except for competitive swimming, they rarely relate it to a strenuous workout. As you'll learn, however, when you change the setting to the deep end of the pool, things can get intense. This intensity is a direct result of buoyancy, density, viscosity, resistance, hydrostatic pressure, turbulence, and drag—important concepts and characteristics that are responsible for the merits of HIT.

WHEN BUOYANCY WORKS, GRAVITY TAKES A BREAK

Deep water fitness is different—it isn't at all like working on land. On land, you have 100% gravity at work. In deep water training, there are virtually no impact forces from gravity. As you move into water up to your pelvis or chest, you'll feel only about 40% to 60% of the effects of gravity. When submerged up to your neck, as you would be in performing deep water interval training, the effect of gravity decreases to 10%, or about 15 pounds (the approximate weight of your own head).[24] According to an article in *Military Medicine*, "Deep water running provides for decreased stress and weight bearing to injured tissue and joints, allows for maintenance of cardiovascular fitness ... and offers greater specificity of exercise, thereby potentially serving as a more optimal alternative exercise than biking or swimming."[25] The minimization of gravity's effect allows you to choose what you want to do on a wide spectrum. No matter what level of intensity you choose, you're minimizing the impact on joints and the potential muscle damage that can happen with land-based fitness.[26] That's why working in water is the perfect modality.

I thought water workouts weren't real workouts—not hard enough. Not to mention I thought I'd look dumb doing them. If you're thinking that right now—stop—because, oh, how wrong I was. If my body is super tight and sore, the water helps me loosen up and recover much faster. If I'm frustrated or just tense, I run for the pool. With even a 20-minute workout of Punches and Cross-Country, I typically get out laughing and feeling like me again. I've been happily addicted to hydro for three years now!

About six months after I first started hydro, a medical situation arose that stumped doctors as my symptoms continued to worsen. It got to the point that I was in severe pain; it hurt to even walk, let alone run, cycle, or box. I was told to back off on everything, but I was still allowed to do hydro training. I adjusted the workouts for how my body felt that day and still feel healthy and in shape.

My health issues have abated and I'm currently training for a marathon with a team. While training for the marathon, I had to have surgery and wasn't able to work out for over a month but, once I got the doctor's clearance, I resumed workouts with water training routines then jumped right back into land running. Now when my teammates are hurting, I teach them water workouts. I talk about it all the time because I LOVE IT! Hydro has been a game changer for me. Now I'm sharing its tremendous benefits with other runners on my team.

—Nichole, runner, land and water boxer, aerospace engineer

Buoyancy is the "lifting" effect or the upward force a body experiences in water; it's the force that makes the body float.[27] This property, most prevalent in water, makes functional, comfortable, and effective no-impact exercise possible. When the human body is immersed in water, the degree of buoyancy is determined by the density of the body in relation to the density of water, and to the amount of water that it displaces. Buoyancy can also be described as a force that counteracts the effects of gravity, which works to pull us toward the ground. So when exercising in water, remember that:

- a body fully immersed up to the neck will displace more water than if you were immersed only to the waist, thus optimizing the positive effects of buoyancy

- a human body that is slim and very muscular is more dense and won't float as much as a larger body, so more than one flotation device may be needed
- a larger body that has a higher percentage of fat is less dense and will float better (i.e., stay higher in the water than the average person) so no flotation device may be required[28]

My husband's recovery from a severely sprained ankle illustrates the exceptional benefits of buoyancy. Any sort of land-based medial or lateral standing ankle exercise was too difficult on his injured ankle. However, he could start recovering in the shallow end of the pool by doing lateral ankle hops as well as maintain his musculature and cardiovascular fitness with continued deep water training. Just a few months later, he was beside me on a 50k trail run in the Santa Cruz Mountains.

Because of the body's full immersion, deep water training also involves learning a new center of gravity (CG). Your body's center of gravity is the point at which your weight is evenly distributed in all directions, making you feel stable and balanced. When moving, the center of gravity adjusts so a healthy, normally functioning body remains upright and avoids falling over. This land-based CG is located around the hips/pelvis region. In water, where gravity is not a factor during movement, this point of balance shifts higher, closer to the chest, and is referred to as center of buoyancy (CB).[29] This shift in location requires a recalibration of body awareness and sense of balance. It may seem unusual to refer to balance in the water setting because the feet aren't on the ground but, because HIT involves specific postural alignment, there can be an adjustment period before mastering the upright position. Some may truly be challenged with this, especially when in motion, even to the point of losing their balance and doing a face plant in the water!

Density plays another very significant role in deep water training when paired with viscosity. Both concepts are primarily responsible for the most integral component of HIT: resistance. As the Aquatic Exercise Association (AEA) states, "Because the water offers resistance, even more force or energy is required to initiate and change movement."[30] Water is about 800 times denser than air, which is in part the cause of resistance; it's the reason that the faster you move in water, the more difficult it feels.[31] Imagine an entire fitness program of working against constant resistance in every direction, resisting each movement of every part of the body. This would be similar to running with multiple elastic bands attached to your limbs, all pulling at different angles. This is what you'll experience with HIT.

Viscosity can be described as the "thickness" experienced when moving in a liquid.[32] Air has very little thickness when compared to water, which is why movements of the unloaded limbs can be so easily carried out on land as opposed to underwater. This quality of water creates a platform that can work to your advantage in exercise because, as you encounter the viscosity of water, a resistance is experienced.

Because movements are also slower than on land, individuals watching from the pool deck often get the impression that a deep water workout is easy, but this is definitely not the case. What the untrained eye doesn't see are the forces working under the surface and the energy and intensity it takes to move one's limbs through the water.

The discussion of viscosity and density leads to another fundamental characteristic of water-based movement: drag. In deep water training, drag is the force that acts against the limbs moving through the water, creating a "heaviness." The term "resistance" refers to this heavy feeling. Drag is boosted when the leading surface area is larger. Simply put, you create more drag when you move an open hand (more surface area) through water than a fisted hand (less surface area). In addition, because of the relationship of speed to drag, the effort needed to push or pull water will increase exponentially as the limb is moved faster.[33]

With the addition of turbulence, drag is accentuated, requiring even more muscle engagement to control the body and move the limbs while exercising. The turbulence in a pool is generated by water current—not from tides, but from your own movement or a fellow participant's movement, either close by or as far as adjacent lanes. A HIT drill that specifically takes advantage of turbulence is the Eddy (page 95), in which participants repeatedly Water Run one direction for about five seconds, then quickly turn 180 degrees and run back into their own water current. With higher levels of turbulence created by everyone doing the movement, the body experiences much higher levels of drag, especially when turning and holding an upright position. The equivalent on land? I consider this to be like a one-minute threshold run in the wind, while moving uphill and going around other runners.

The amazing part of water, though, is that as soon as you stop moving, almost all forces (except for buoyancy) cease as well.

HYDROSTATIC PRESSURE

Water is dense and, because of gravity, heavy—just over 8 pounds per gallon. Fill an entire pool and it becomes an enormous amount of weight. The weight of the water that envelopes the body is what causes hydrostatic pressure (HP). In fact, the deeper a person is submerged, the greater the HP will be exerting its force on the body. Deep-sea and scuba divers are very familiar with this phenomenon. It's hard to conceptualize because you don't feel different when you enter the water. Yet, when submerged to your chest or neck, this pressure compresses your body and contributes to the resistance to movement.[34] Think of how this pressure would affect your respiratory muscles, even more than land-based training. When you breathe in, your muscles need to expand your lungs and rib cage. In water, those same muscles must work harder against the pressure of the water when taking a breath. Research has found improved athletic performance with increased ease and ability to "breathe during peak exercise levels when returning to land after aquatic exercise."[35]

HOW WATER AFFECTS HEART RATE

Oddly enough, when some athletes are immersed in water to the neck and pushed through a workout program, they may think they're not working hard enough because of their lower heart rates (HR) compared to when exercising on land. This is one of the major reasons athletes avoid using the pool as an acceptable option for cross-training. They feel they're not "doing enough." There are many components involved in the effect of the heart rate running lower in water than during a comparable land-based exercise. This is an important issue to consider given the high intensity levels involved in HIT. However, this discussion can be quite lengthy and technical, so I've chosen to give a brief explanation and then turn my primary focus to how to monitor HR and suggestions for managing effort levels with HIT.

In a two-part round-table discussion by Dr. Gregory Haff, published in *National Strength and Conditioning Association*, Dr. Haff gathered scholars in the field to discuss water-based exercise as a cross-training modality.[36] He asked the scholars questions to shed light on what was known regarding the effects of the immersed body when training. Haff concluded that when a body is immersed, heart rates can be anywhere from 10% to 30% lower due to various effects on the function of the heart, and other experts expressed similar findings.[37] This means that you can train in the water with a lower heart rate but still work as hard as you would on land. Therefore, it's important to understand how to make adjustments for this lowered heart rate. For details on how to calculate your aquatic heart rate, see Finding Your HIT Target Heart Rate for Water Exercise on page 83.

WATER TEMPERATURE & HIT

Water temperature can significantly influence comfort in the pool and enjoyment of water exercise. Therefore, understanding the basics of how water temperature affects participants is extremely valuable. Even with this knowledge, optimal pool temperature can be something of a challenge, especially if it's not in your control. The two main points to consider in determining the best temperature are the intensity of the workout and the level to which the body is immersed in the water.

Competitive swimmers will say the optimal water temperature should be between 78° and 82° but, if you ask anyone using the pool for aqua aerobics, water yoga, rehabilitation, arthritis, or lupus, this water temperature is too cold.[38] Circulation slows with the cooler temperatures, and blood flow lessens in the extremities and is directed more to the trunk region, where the major organs are located.[39] These less-intense workouts in shallow water require warmer temperatures for general comfort, to reduce risk of excessive heat loss, and to gain some relief from joint discomforts and stiffness. However, during hydro interval training or swimming, both vigorous high-intensity interval workouts that generate increased blood flow throughout the body, the circulatory effects of cooler water are overcome, and lower temperatures are required. The following chart[40] gives a guideline as to which water temperature works best with different types of water activities:

WATER ACTIVITY	COLD 50–59°F (10–15°C)	COOL 78.8–84.2°F (26–29°C)	NEUTRAL 92.3–95.9°F (33.5–35.5°C)	WARM 96.8–101.3°F (36–38.5°C)
Ice baths after exercise	X			
Hot/cold immersion baths	X			X
Vigorous exercise		X		
Arthritis exercise			X	
Typical aquatic therapy			X	
Cardiac rehab			X	
Multiple sclerosis exercise		X		
Spinal cord injury programs			X	
Parkinson's programming			X	
Relaxation				X

Deep water participants can benefit from the increased blood flow of a slightly warmer temperature but, if too warm, the risk of overheating increases. I've found that temperatures above 84° can create overheating, with participants becoming sluggish and excessively perspiring in the body's attempt to cool itself. (Yes, people perspire in the water—you see it on their faces.) Yet, too cold, and you risk potential cramping of the extremities.[41] It's important to note, though, that overheating and overworking can happen in the water even with appropriate pool temperatures, just as it can happen on land.

Over the years, I've found that the best temperature range is 79° to 82°, very similar to the optimum temperature for competitive swimmers. This is because the intensity level of deep water interval work is more strenuous and demanding, and higher temperatures negatively affect exercise tolerance. In this range, it's still warm enough to keep the blood flowing to the extremities, while still utilizing the cooling properties of the water to moderate the increased body heat generated during the strenuous exercise.

Body temperature is affected by the level to which it's immersed simply because the body tends to get cold when it's wet and exposed to ambient temperature or outside breezes. This will happen more often when training in water at waist level since the deeper the body is immersed (as with deep water training), the less exposed it is to outside temperatures. If you feel like you're not warm enough during your workout, wear a water shirt to minimize temperature changes.

As with any fitness program, individualization remains key. If too warm, slow down to stabilize your body temperature. If you're cold, it's likely a problem of function and form. Ask yourself, "Are you performing the strokes correctly?" "Are you working at the indicated intensities?" Typically the answer will be "no." Deep water interval training is not meant to be comfortable and easy. Done right, it will make you work and perspire. This is not your grandma's water aerobics.

PART 2

The Exercises & Program Notes

CHAPTER 4

Let's Get Started: Basic Hand Positions & Strokes

In general, research has shown aquatic exercise to be at least the equivalent in training value to land-based training, which may refute the myth that water exercise isn't an aerobically efficient training method.[42]

Now that you've gotten the fundamentals of deep water training, let's jump into the good stuff—learning the exercises. You may know a move like the Water Run but not recognize its full potential. This chapter will give you the in-depth understanding of the Water Run and other strokes so you can reap the full benefits of deep water exercises. Along with detailed instructions, I've provided advice for training and coaching. There's a learning curve with many of these strokes so be aware that more than one workout may be needed to master the movements. As a coach you'll eventually be able to look down into the water and quickly tell which muscles are being engaged and, most importantly, which ones are not.

Flexibility and range of motion (ROM), or the degree of reach of each limb, varies from person to person. It's important that individuals respect their ROM, which helps to keep their body in proper alignment and promotes balance and core stability, the keys to achieving maximal benefit. An integral component of working in deep water is that it effectively provides the opportunity to readily identify and correct strength, coordination, and movement imbalances.

Training in deep water also magnifies your imbalances so that you can correct and account for them.

—Colter, mountain biker

The exercises are organized into five hand positions and four strokes. The hand positions partner with the strokes to increase or decrease the resistance felt during the exercise, and to change the muscle focus. By practicing the hand positions with the basic Water Run, you'll also learn how viscosity, drag, and buoyancy all affect even the smallest surface area: your hand.

The mechanics of the four basic strokes are fully detailed. When combined with hand positions, the adaptable strokes demonstrate the versatility of deep water training. Each description will include a focused power phase; sometimes it's balanced between both the backward and forward motions, and sometimes emphasis is placed in one direction.

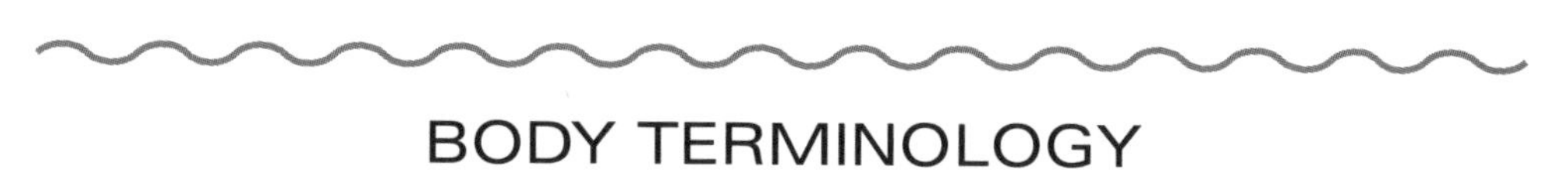

BODY TERMINOLOGY

Here are some terms that are used in the exercise descriptions:

Horizontal (transverse) plane: This imaginary plane, parallel to the ground, horizontally separates your lower and upper body.

Median (midsagittal) plane: The median plane separates the left and right sides of the body.

Frontal (coronal) plane: This plane divides the front and back of the body.

Trunk: Also referred to as the torso, the trunk is the central portion of the body, not including the head, arms, or legs.

Abdominals (abs): The abs are the muscles located in the abdomen (or belly) area.

Upper limbs: This includes your shoulder and arms.

Lower limbs: This includes your hips, buttocks, and legs.

When deep water training, you'll be activating your core muscles, including but not limited to:

- rectus abdominis
- transverse abdominis
- external and internal obliques
- erector spinae and multifidus (lower and middle back)
- gluteals

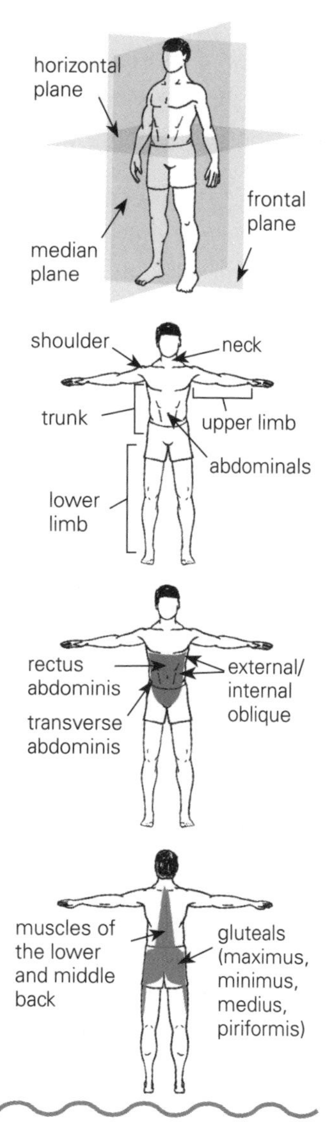

TEST AT HOME

To experience the various effects of different hand positions outside of the pool, put your hand in a sinkful of water and move it around using different strokes. Do this for a minute to get a sense of how the different positions feel; you'll see that each stroke can and will become harder with increased effort.

When the stroke's recovery phase for the limb isn't clarified, it's because the recovery movement pattern is inconsequential. But every stroke discusses core/abdominal involvement and engagement—an important aspect to performing HIT accurately. When the core isn't engaged, the participant struggles with correct form and consequently won't experience the intended benefits. When done right, there's nothing easy about deep water interval training.

Form issues, notes for coaching poolside, terminology, and workout suggestions are all accompanied by both underwater images and views from the deck to fully grasp how the strokes look, even when distorted by the water's movement.

Also provided are PT points and basic tips ranging from cautions to potential contraindications for each move. These are especially important for individuals who are recovering or rehabilitating from injuries or surgeries. The physical therapy components will offer readers another perspective as to the effects of movement and exercise, as well as educate and assist in sound body care and awareness.

HAND POSITIONS

Hand positions affect the overall movement of any stroke. Changing the hand position to work with or against the water's resistance and drag is crucial in customizing a workout. In fact, adjusting the hand position is one of the most basic ways someone can make a workout harder or easier. Modifying the angle or finger position changes the drag generated by the hand moving through the water, increasing or decreasing the overall effort for any given stroke. These small changes can even be used to affect which muscle groups are targeted.

The first four hand positions will be demonstrated with the Water Run. By describing the entire arm movement, you'll learn how to perform and incorporate the hand positions in this basic move. Once you master the Water Run using the various hand positions, you can apply that knowledge to other strokes. The fifth hand position is utilized in just two strokes.

General PT points. When the arm is pulled through the water, some of the hand positions generate increased drag, placing stronger forces on the elbow and shoulder joints. If you disregard your form, you increase the possibility of straining anywhere from your wrist to your neck. Make sure you follow the detailed descriptions of the arm movements. Regardless of the intensity of the exercise, never lock out your elbow joint for any stroke—it creates excessive forces on the joints. Shoulder injuries or conditions that require extra precautions include (but aren't limited to):

- Rotator cuff injury/surgery
- Shoulder reconstruction
- Shoulder dislocation, impingement, tendinitis, or bursitis
- Recent fracture

Hand positions and injuries. Occasionally when working with people post-shoulder/arm injuries, the use of any hand position, even with a low effort level, may place too much force on the shoulder. In these cases, avoid using the arms altogether. To do so, place your arms across the torso or on the hips for any exercise that agitates the upper body in a painful way. Be prepared for a harder core workout—no arm movement increases the need for core stabilization as the arms are no longer providing a counter force for the leg motion.

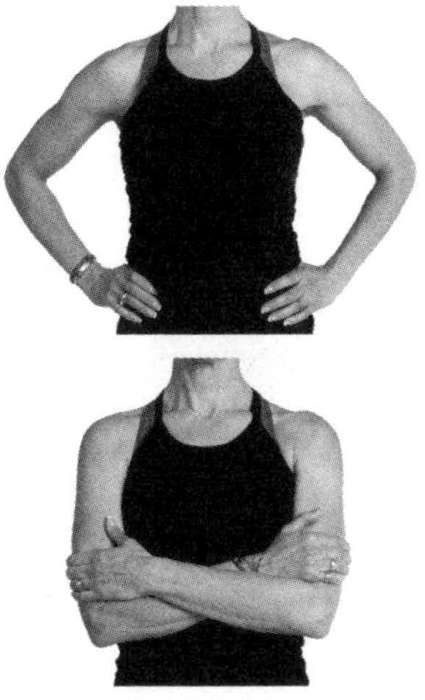

If you are not using a hand position, place your arms on your waist or across your torso.

OPEN HAND

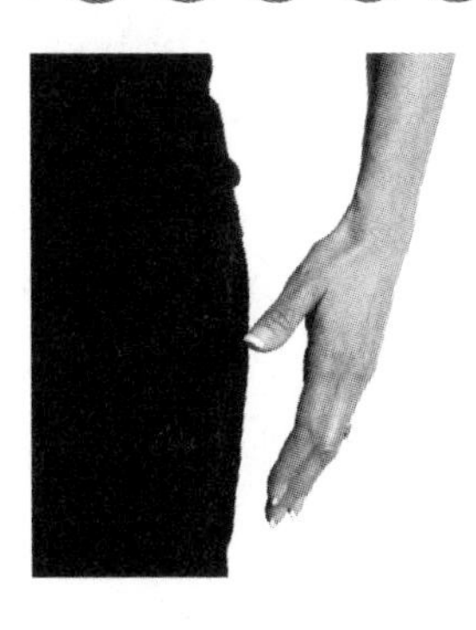

Used in a majority of deep water exercises, the Open Hand position serves as a paddle to create the driving force. An Open Hand displaces more water when pulling, which produces a more forceful arm stroke.

To start, hold your hand palm down and flat (parallel to the surface of the water) with fingers lightly held together. When used in a Water Run, the palm faces downward toward the pool floor. Only the thumb and pointer finger should brush lightly against your body as you push your arm down and back during the arm motion.

FORM ISSUES

A novice mistake is stiffening the hand, which is a natural response when first experiencing water pressure against your body. Don't stiffen your open hands! This causes a chain reaction of rigidity moving from the hands to the wrists, elbows, and shoulders, stiffening the entire arm movement. If this occurs, relax your hands and arms.

PT POINTS

Increased pressure is put at the wrist joint to keep the wrist from bending backward against the force of the water. When an Open Hand position combines with a straighter arm, it works like a long lever, applying even more force on your joints. Levers are great for lifting heavy things but not so great on the joints if your muscles haven't developed the strength to support them sufficiently. Also make sure to avoid a locked-out elbow. When pulling through the arm stroke, a scooping action of the hand and wrist can lead to excessive stress and strain on those joints as well as the forearm muscles. If you notice scooping, correct this error promptly by relaxing your hand. Wrist injuries or conditions that require extra precautions include (but aren't limited to):

- Carpal tunnel syndrome/surgery
- Tendinitis in the elbow or shoulder
- Medial epicondylitis, more commonly known as golfer's or tennis elbow
- Recent fractures

PARTIALLY OPEN

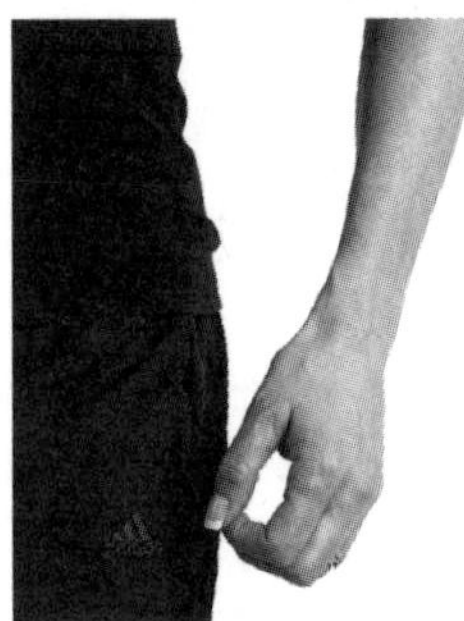

This position is similar to the Open Hand but the difference is that the hand is relaxed with the pointer finger and thumb touching or almost touching each other. I sometimes jokingly refer to this position as a "tea cup" hand (as when drinking tea "properly" with the thumb and first four fingers and the pinky finger almost raised). The drag produced from the partially open hand allows a runner to engage more of their upper body, though the effects are not as great as with the flat Open Hand position.

When used with the Water Run, the arm goes through the same path as the Open Hand position but with the wrists slightly rotated toward the hips. This rotation makes the thumb and all the fingertips brush the hips when performing the stroke. I find that this hand position works best for runners doing deep water exercises; it simulates the same position when running on land. The stroke can also promote a relaxed upper body, which counteracts the stiffness that sometimes happens with an Open or Closed Hand position (page 31).

FORM ISSUES

As with the Open Hand position, participants may generate stiffness and rigidity in their joints when pulling through the stroke. Scooping with the hand/wrist on the pull-through of the stroke is a potential problem if you're used to quickly traveling through the water with paddle-effect of the Open Hand. Since a Partially Open Hand produces less drag (thus less propulsion), you may compensate by trying to create more power through scooping. Don't! It's okay that you're moving through the water at a slower speed. It's more important to keep your wrists relaxed.

PT POINTS

The Partially Open Hand generates the same forces on the wrist joint as the Open Hand (see page 31) but to a lesser degree, and could be used as a modification for the Open Hand to decrease resistance and intensity.

CLOSED HAND

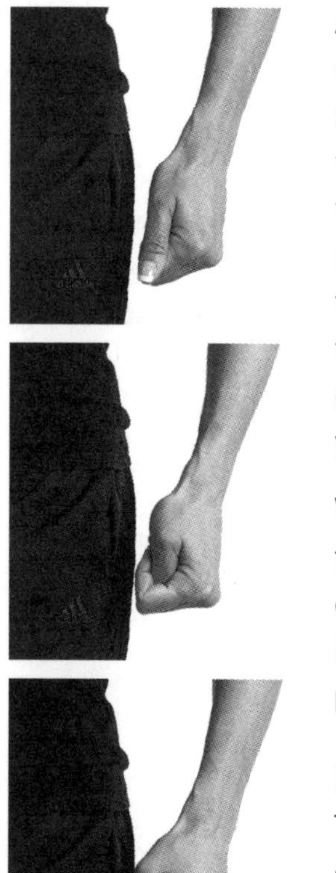

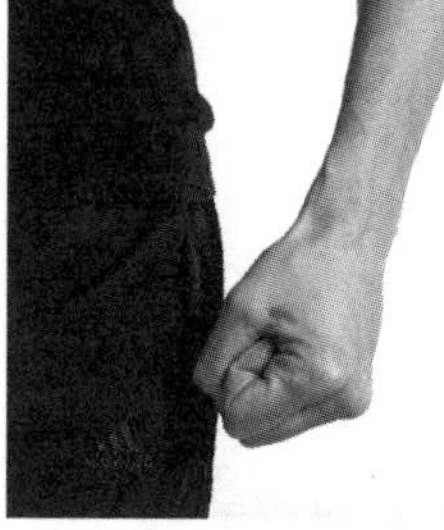

A Closed Hand is basically a loosely held fist. Gently close your hand—don't clench it closed because that will tighten the elbow and shoulder and potentially lock your arms. This hand position forces you to drive through your core more because the trunk muscles (particularly the transverse abdominals) need to work harder to find stability when the hand position no longer provides it. This is a good hand position to use when you can't get the hang of engaging your entire arm through to the core as the reduced drag of the Closed Hand position can facilitate abdominal engagement. Drills that use a Closed Hand position intensify the use of your core.

When using the Closed Hand in a Water Run, the insides of the wrists face toward the body. When driving through the stroke, the backs of the curled fingers brush past the hips. The thumb can be tucked into the hand, held in front/on top of the fingers, or even rest on the first finger—it's a personal choice.

FORM ISSUES

The Closed Hand position can be frustrating—it doesn't generate the same drag as the Open Hand so there's also a tendency to scoop the hand/wrist when driving through an arm swing. Be sure to not scoop the hand or wrist.

PT POINTS

With the Closed Hand position, the arm moves more easily and quickly through the water. This is desirable for reducing stress on the shoulder, elbow, and wrist joints.

If you still feel shoulder discomfort or pain, decrease the speed and/or range of the motion until sufficient muscle conditioning develops and/or sufficient recovery takes place.

SLICING HAND

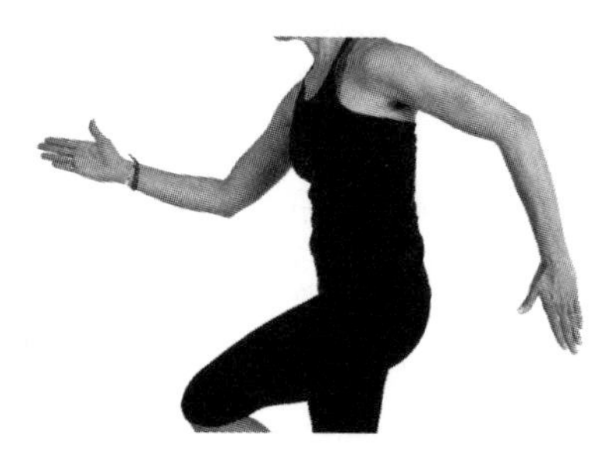

The Slicing Hand position creates the least amount of drag of all the hand positions. In fact, there's so little that it's unnoticeable (as the only drag is from the arm itself). It's ideal for those working through shoulder issues—less resistance means the arm and shoulder area exerts less effort.

To start, extend your right arm out with your hand flat but palm facing the left toward your midline. Perform the arm movement by moving the arm down as if cutting through the water. The position has very little drag and therefore may facilitate more core engagement (similar to what happens with the Closed Hand). This increases the demands of the trunk muscles for intense conditioning and strengthening.

I found after my bike accident (both times landing on my right shoulder going over 30 miles an hour) that the Open Hand or Partial Hand created too much muscle activation in my shoulder. The Slicing Hand allowed my arm to drive through the movement without drag—the perfect rehabilitation movement until my shoulder strength improved.

FORM ISSUES

The most common problem is rigid hands caused by stiffened wrists. This rigidity causes the elbow then the shoulder to stiffen. Keep the wrist loose.

PT POINTS

The Slicing Hand position has the same concerns as the Closed Hand position. See PT Points on page 33.

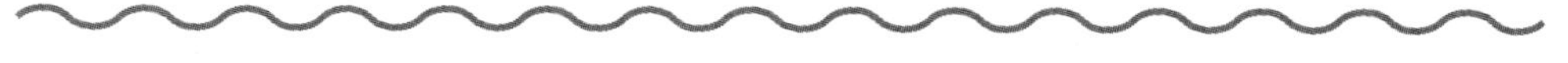

ANATOMY OF A STROKE

Catch: the initiation or start of the stroke

Power phase: the part of the stroke that generates the most effort

Recovery phase: the part of the stroke that's the least effort

Pull: describes when the stroke is moving toward the body only; similar to power phase

Follow-through: when a limb moves through to the end of the intended range of motion for any particular stroke

REVERSE HAND

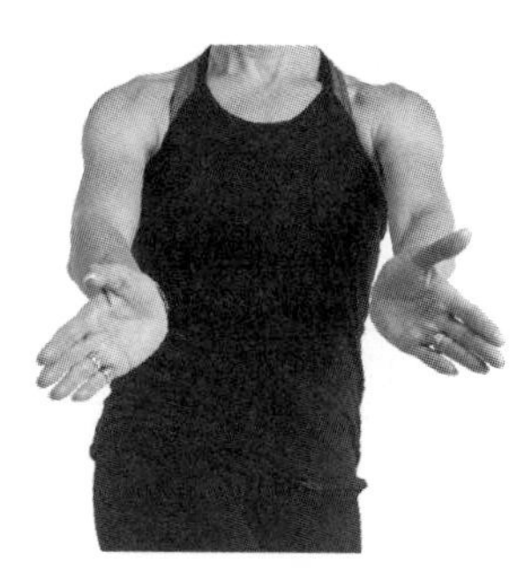

The Reverse Hand isn't used frequently; in fact it's performed with just two exercises, the Water Walk and Breast Stroke. The Reverse Hand motion drastically changes the focus point of the engaged muscles, significantly changing the stroke.

To perform, rotate your arms inward so that your palms face each other and the *back* of the hands lead the stroke and pull through the water. Please review the Reverse Water Walk (page 57) and the Reverse Breast Stroke (page 64) for full understanding of the use of this hand position.

FORM ISSUES

Watch out for a locked wrist and raised/shrugged shoulders when using this hand position with the Reverse Water Walk. An overreaching arm is common with the Reverse Breast Stroke. See the Form Issues sections of the Reverse Water Walk (page 57) and Reverse Breast Stroke (page 64) for further details.

PT POINTS

The Reverse Hand puts increased pressure on the wrist joint in order to prevent the wrist from bending forward against the force of the water. The muscles responsible for this action are smaller and usually weaker than the stabilizer wrist muscles used in the Open Hand position. Pay attention to pain and/or fatigue in these smaller muscles that control the wrist. Conditions that require extra precautions include (but aren't limited to):

- Lateral epicondylitis, more commonly known as tennis elbow
- Carpal tunnel

See PT Points for Reverse Water Walk (page 58) and the Reverse Breast Stroke (page 65) for important shoulder precautions when using this hand position.

HOW TO INSTRUCT FROM THE DECK

Instruction for all the hand positions are similar. In most cases, frequent reminders are necessary to point out what the hand position should feel like (relaxed but engaged) and what should be avoided (scooping or a tightening of the wrist). General group reminders may suffice, but work individually with those participants who are having trouble.

Reinforce your verbal instructions by demonstrating the correct form. Remember, there are no mirrors, so they can't "see" what they're doing. When demonstrating, move through the arm/hand motion slowly, describing each phase of the hand position being performed. Show the group your hand in proper form, then have them move their own arms.

It's helpful to shift back and forth from one hand stroke to another to highlight subtle differences. For example, compare the Partially Open Hand with the Open Hand and explain how less drag creates more core engagement and vice versa. I also talk about the Slicing and Closed hands together, reminding the group that these two hand positions produce the least amount of drag, so they'll need to produce more stability through their core to maintain proper full-body form. The more you communicate with clients on what they should be feeling, the better!

Keep your coaching flexible based on what you see in the pool. If participants are using an Open Hand position but are pulling with just their hands, I'll switch to a Closed Hand stroke in the middle of a set to bring about core engagement. When this happens, remind the participants about feeling the increased core engagement and to be mindful of not scooping.

Useful terms and phrases include:

- Keep your shoulders relaxed.
- Hands loose, not stiff.
- Increase your core engagement.

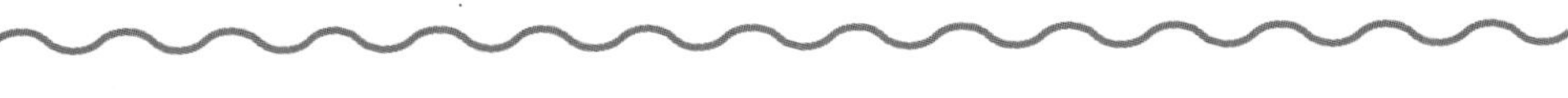

FIRST-TIME DEEP WATER INSTRUCTORS

If you've never coached deep water exercises before, your success will improve tremendously if you personally experiment with the strokes and experience all the effects of deep water on body motion. One mistake first-timers make is demonstrating the strokes too quickly. When you do the actual moves in water, you become aware of the water's viscosity and will learn to demonstrate proper form more slowly when on deck, as if you're physically in the water. And always remember that communication is important in both teaching the stroke and helping the person become aware of where the body is at any given time.

HOW TO USE HAND POSITIONS IN A WORKOUT

Once you understand the hand positions, it's simple to interchange them within a routine. Choose a main stroke (such as the Water Run) and a starting hand position. Then change the hand positions over the workout's duration, which gives participants a taste of how just changing the hand position can manipulate a workout to increase or decrease difficulty. A simple series is to use the hand position with the most drag (Open Hand) and finish the position with the least drag (Slicing Hand). This progression will effectively show how you engage your core more as you generate less drag with your hands.

Changing hand positions is also helpful when focusing on core engagement. If you find you are not engaging your core enough with an Open Hand, change to a Closed Hand or Slicing Hand, which puts the focus on engaging the core. A good way to cycle through different hand positions is with a 1-minute progressive Water Run Drill:

- 20 seconds Open Hand at 75% effort,
- 20 seconds Partially Open Hand at 80% effort,
- 20 seconds, Closed Hand or a Slicing Hand at 85% effort.

Rest 30 seconds before repeating the sequence. Do 5 repetitions. Total time is 7.5 minutes.

For a full explanation on how to customize a workout, see Chapter 6.

BASIC DEEP WATER STROKES

Now that you understand the five hand positions, we can delve into the four main strokes. (Chapter 5 details 16 more advanced strokes and variations.) Several strokes have similar details repeated. This is intentional—repeating the important reminders for each will help when referring back to a specific stroke, as you'll have the information you need at your fingertips.

The limbs power every stroke. Unlike shallow-water or land-based exercises that connect to a grounding force (closed kinetic chain), the freedom of simultaneous leg and arm motions in deep water allows for a wide variability in movements and also requires increased muscle stability throughout the body.

There are generally two types of leg motions that drive the strokes. The first uses a straighter line of motion with a straighter knee (e.g., Cross-Country, Water Walk, Flutter Kick) while the second uses vigorous leg action with increased knee flexion (e.g., Breast Stroke, Water Run, High Knee, Karate Kick). If you need to limit knee flexion or want a more restrained leg motion, there will be numerous choices to meet your needs.

While the strokes have parallel names to some land activities, the pool environment is vastly different than exercising on land. Moving the body while immersed in water in a specific, intended manner requires conscious attention and experimentation, especially in the early learning stages. You'll need to develop a new kinesthetic (body) awareness that requires a heightened level of concentration. Because there are no mirrors and no realistic way for an instructor to physically move clients into the correct form, the best way to instruct is through clear verbal and physical demonstrations from the deck. If you're learning this on your own, the "trial and error" method eventually pays off.

WATER RUN

When people think of deep water exercising, they think of the Water Run. This is a fundamental stroke that sets the foundation for the rest of the strokes. This iconic movement requires a tall spine, shoulders anchored down by the muscles in the back, and an engaged core—form that's necessary for *all* interval training in the water.

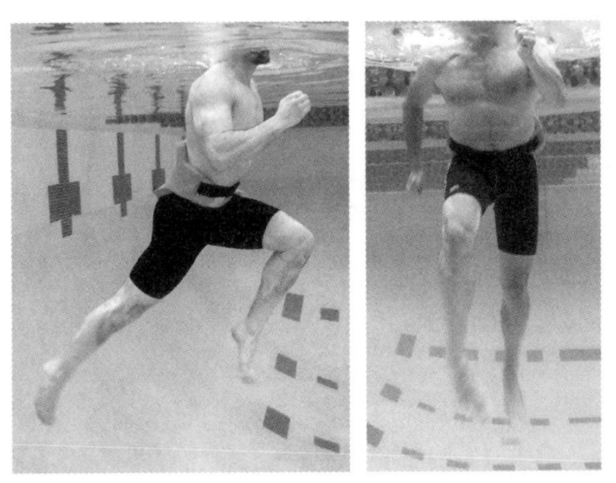

Correct Water Run form.

To begin in the pool, position your body vertically with a slight forward lean. The arms and legs move the same as on land: Right arm and left leg move forward first; as they return to the starting position, the left arm and right leg move forward in a continuous flow. The power phase of this stroke comes from the limbs moving from the front position to the back position. The head and chin are above water but, in some cases, the chin (and occasionally the mouth) may dip temporarily into the water. If the chin/mouth is under the water, make sure it's simply due to the greater body density of the runner rather than a body position that's leaning too far forward. This may seem obvious, but over the years I've actually witnessed people sinking underwater for extended periods of time while holding their breath in a Water Run. Don't do this! Additional flotation may be necessary for a person who can't stay above the water. Be sure you're able to take regular breaths safely by keeping your mouth and chin above the water the majority of the time. (See Tools of the Trade on page 13 for more on flotation devices and body density.)

While similar to its land counterpart, the Water Run is slightly different. The most notable distinction is that the open kinetic chain of deep water exercise uncovers core instabilities immediately, whereas on land this may not be noticeable. The range of motion for the Water Run's leg stroke is similar on land, including:

- Foot dorsiflexion (foot/toes pointed upward) when the knee rises and the leg advances forward

- Foot plantarflexion (foot/toes pointed downward), with a slight scoop of the foot as the leg extends down and back when pulling through the stroke
- Use of the quadriceps when bringing the leg forward and up while extending the knee
- Use of the hamstrings and glutes during the follow-through of the stroke.

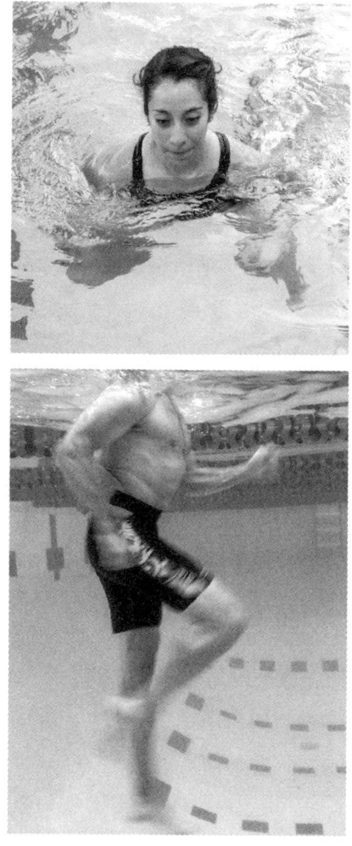

Incorrect: Top image shows legs too far apart and lower image shows person too straight with no forward lean. Both reduce the stroke's effectiveness.

Let go of any expectations that you'll travel through the water at the same pace as on land; you'll be slower. Even with high effort, you'll be going slowly through the pool. Typically, a land runner who tries the Water Run for the first time will erroneously move the legs in more of a high step or march, or almost like running over hurdles. This may be partially due to the lack of coordination that's initially experienced or because they are trying to Water Run at a cadence they're accustomed to on land before they've learned how to engage the proper muscles.

I frequently incorporate the legs-only Water Run in workouts, which promotes increased hamstring work since there's no upper body to help propel a runner through the water. The main reason to remove the use of the upper body for the Water Run (or any of the strokes) is to promote better lower-body movement and to induce core engagement. By isolating the leg motion and narrowing the focus, participants may find it easier to work on a specific weak area or a particularly challenging form component.

Doing the legs-only Water Run also helps individuals master the leg motion. I've seen some very accomplished runners enter the water, only to have their bodies crumple before me; hips thrust behind them, legs spinning like they're on a tricycle, elbows pointing out and arms pumping in tight little arcs ending about six inches in front of their hips (aka T-rexing). Isolating the legs assists the transition to proper body alignment, complete core engagement, and improved leg motion. Once this is accomplished, arm movements can be reintroduced.

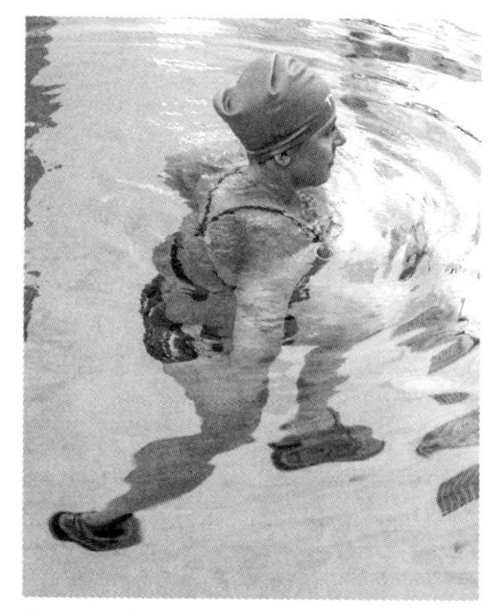

Correct legs-only Water Run.

A good arm swing strengthens the arms, back, and core, all of which help a runner produce more power when on land. Using different hand positions during the Water Run affects how much or how little intensity the movement has. To start, I'll use the Partial Hand position to demonstrate the Water Run arm swing.

Start the arm swing with the elbow at a 90-degree angle. The hand/arm will move up and forward to about 6 to 8 inches below the surface of the water, and then swing back with the arm driving down past the hips, the thumb and tips of the index and middle fingers brushing slightly against the hips. The hand finishes at or just behind the hips, producing a slight elbow extension. Regardless of which hand position is being used, the hand would stay in the same position as it returns to the forward position. During this stroke, the arm swing forward would actually be the countereffect to the opposite leg moving up (just as it would be on land).

The Water Run works the core, quads, hamstrings, glutes, calves, upper arms, and back. Focus on turning the legs over at a cadence similar to your running cadence on land (without losing form, as mentioned earlier). Hitting your land-based running cadence in the water may have you at sprinting intensities since it works more muscles. The arm stroke matches the effort of the legs—the harder or faster the legs move, the harder or faster the countering upper body performs in like rhythm. I'll frequently cue my students, "Equal upper-body strokes to lower-body strokes."

FORM ISSUES

Uncoordinated limb movements. Initially, the counter-limb movement is difficult for some people who want to move their limbs on the same side of the body at the same time. Try swinging your right arm and leg forward at the same time. Awkward, isn't it? Yet, you'll see new participants do this every time. This is what full-body immersion in water and the open kinetic chain does; it distorts your ability to sense where your limbs are and how they're moving when attempting to replicate a very familiar movement. Swimmers transitioning to deep water training manifest their own imbalances. Swimmers often want to move their legs more quickly than their upper bodies, as they'd naturally do swimming freestyle.

Traveling too quickly. In deep water running, moving more quickly through the water doesn't always equate to being fitter or stronger. It actually often means that you're either excessively pulling or scooping through the stroke with the hands and wrists instead of also using the full surface of the arm or you're not effectively balancing the stroke by driving the arm to the back position, or you're not correctly driving the arm completely to the back position. This hand/wrist scoop will also place more force on the forearm muscles and has the potential to aggravate an elbow and/or promote wrist or elbow tendinitis. To encourage moving more slowly and taking full advantage of the resistance, recall that the main objective of HIT is to work all body parts equally against the water resistance!

Excessive body lean. When you lean too far forward, you use almost a dog paddle stroke to propel your body through the water more quickly than it should. When you lean back, you're unable to perform the entire follow-through of the stroke, missing out on the strengthening benefits for the hamstrings, glutes, and core. I always have fun demonstrating this as I usually get a good laugh when I mimic a forward or backward lean.

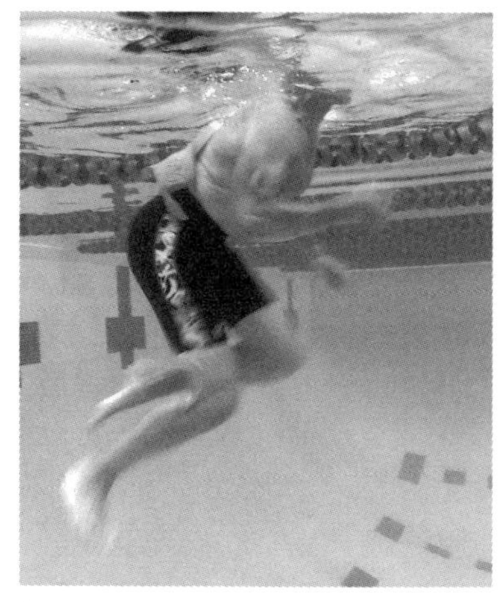

Incorrect: excessive forward body lean, hip hitching, and T-rexing.

Hitching at the hips. This appears as though the rear/hips are resting on a bench, knees moving only up and down without the scooping action, which engages mostly the quadriceps and not the hamstrings. Because the legs are not fully lengthened and stay bent through the hips, the leg is unable to swing through a full range of motion forward or backward. This happens with both experienced and inexperienced people, and is more prominent when participants become tired and their form begins to fall apart.

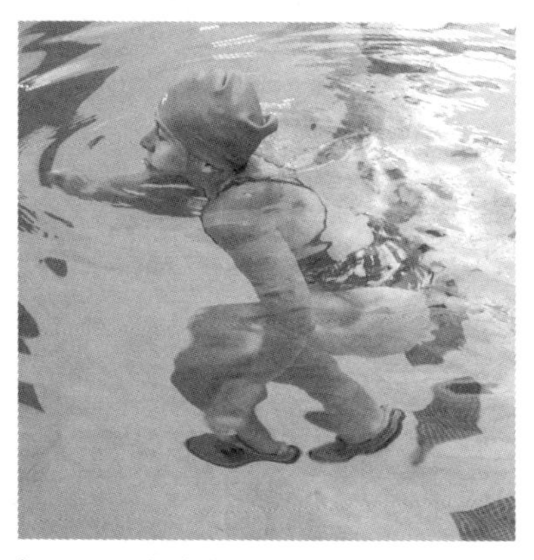

Incorrect belt-less run with hip hitch and T-rex arms.

When the Water Run is performed correctly, there should be a point at which the leg disappears from view if one were to look straight down. If hitching, both legs will be visible the entire time! It can be a bit tricky to correct. An instructor can mimic the incorrect form from the deck (again, there will be laughter) and then remind participants of the proper position. Ask the participant to reach a bit more forward as well as a bit farther behind them than their normal ROM for this stroke (I refer to it as an "outstretched run"), especially focusing on the limbs powering behind the body. Have the group slowly quicken the cadence and shorten the stroke back to their normal ROM, while reminding them to maintain the same muscle engagement of their hamstrings and triceps. A drill of five 1 minute progressive sets of this action may correct the stride.

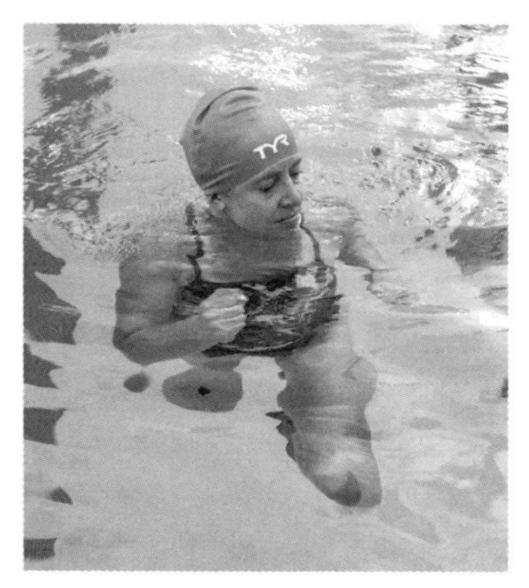

Incorrect: T-rexing

Locked hand or arms. Watch to see if you notice scooping with a stiffened wrist or a rigid positioning of the arm (it's very noticeable—think of plastic dolls that have arms bent at the elbow and how they move; the movement will look the same!). Remind participants about relaxing and not locking their hands or arms.

Incorrect arm motion, aka T-rexing. This occurs when participants don't move their arms through a full range of motion, usually stopping about 6 inches before their hips rather than just slightly after the hips. The shoulders may be raised and the arms may also stay high, almost in a "fighter's" stance (protecting the torso). I refer to this as T-rexing because it looks like a Tyrannosaurus rex's small arms flailing. This can happen any time a person does a Water Run using any hand position, and typically when individuals become tired and form begins to fall apart. To correct, have the participants start into a Water Run (any hand position) but cue for them to feel their fingers brush past their hips. Both focusing on this motion and feeling the sensation across the hips will help with the kinesthetic awareness of where their arms should be.

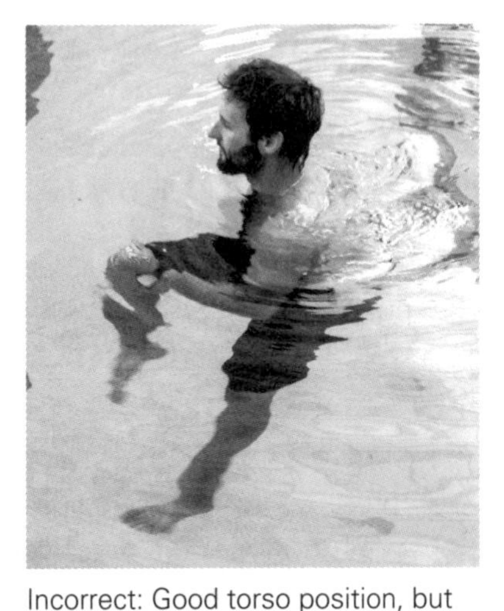

Incorrect: Good torso position, but legs too far forward.

PT POINTS

If hitching at the hips occurs with the hips and lower spine drifting up and backward, the core muscles aren't maintaining the proper body alignment of the trunk and hips. The vigorous leg movement and the misaligned position of the body can strain the lower back. Correct the hitching as soon as possible.

When the leg stroke is going backward, the foot scoops, strongly engaging the calf muscles and the hamstrings at the back of the thigh. If you've had a recent hamstring injury, this movement may be uncomfortable. To adjust this motion, decrease the power of the knee bending action as the leg moves backward. If your hamstring or calf muscle cramps, immediately straighten the leg out in front with the toes/foot flexed upward to stretch out the muscles. Use the side of the pool for added support and stabilization while stretching.

HOW TO INSTRUCT FROM THE DECK

I demonstrate this and other strokes by standing with one leg planted while moving the other limbs. If you need to steady yourself with one hand as well, demonstrate with the arm and leg of the same side. By demonstrating the motions without actually running in place, you can show the slight lean, the full arm swing moving past the hips, and the scoop of the legs. Mimic the pace desired (using a typical warm-up to interval cadence) while simultaneously describing each part of the stroke being performed. Also demonstrate what it looks like when the arm doesn't move past the hip by holding the arms closer to the body (a "fighter's" stance) and not swinging to or past the hips (i.e., "T-rexing").

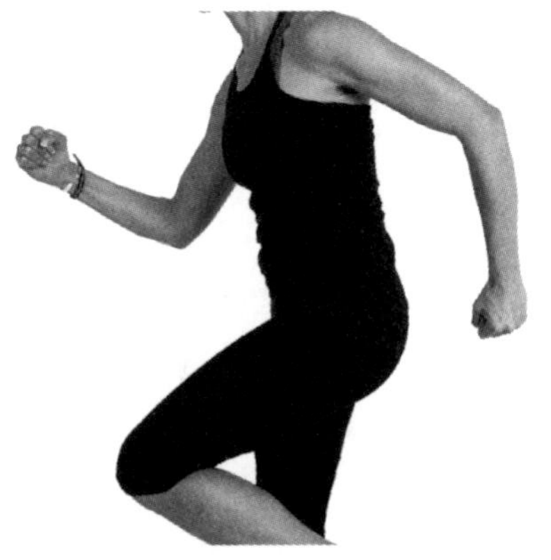

Demonstrating the Water Run with Closed Hands.

Over the years I've found that matching an average participant's limb speed during my demonstrations will help all individuals relate to the motion. In typical water running demonstrations done on land, the instructor will run more quickly in place, leaving participants attempting to match the speed but, due to water resistance, failing. This will create unnecessary frustration.

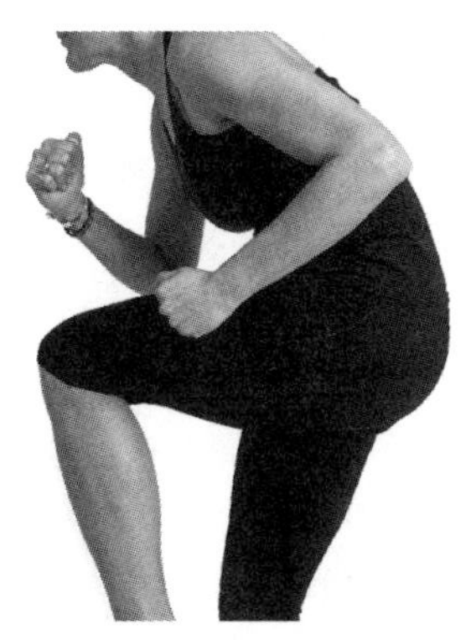

Demonstrating incorrect T-rex arms and hip hitching.

NOTE: In every new group there will be a participant who'll attempt to do whatever stroke you're demonstrating exactly as you're demonstrating it—with just three limbs moving. Therefore, remind the participants that you're not Peter Pan and can't demonstrate with all four limbs!

Remember that when in a pool, the participants can't check their form. Frequent demonstrations and verbal cues are exactly what they need. Therefore, during the demonstrations, describe what they should be feeling and how they should be moving. If needed, isolate the stroke by showing just the lower-body or just the upper-body motion. Useful terms and phrases include:

- Remember to stay relaxed while increasing your effort.
- Hold your body with a slight lean forward.
- Engage through the core.
- Focus on your hamstrings. Feel them pull through the water. (The latter is for those who are hitching and only driving their knees up and down.)
- Follow-through on the arm swing—no T-rexing!

HOW TO USE THE WATER RUN IN A WORKOUT

One way I like to use the Water Run in a workout is to highlight the different hand positions by cycling though one position every 15 seconds, progressively working harder each 15 seconds, totaling 45 seconds or a minute for each set. For a full explanation on how to customize a workout, see Chapter 6.

CROSS-COUNTRY

In the Cross-Country, the upper and lower limbs reach farther than in the Water Run. This promotes even greater strength gains of the core and the upper and lower limbs, as well as increased range of motion of the hips and torso rotation.

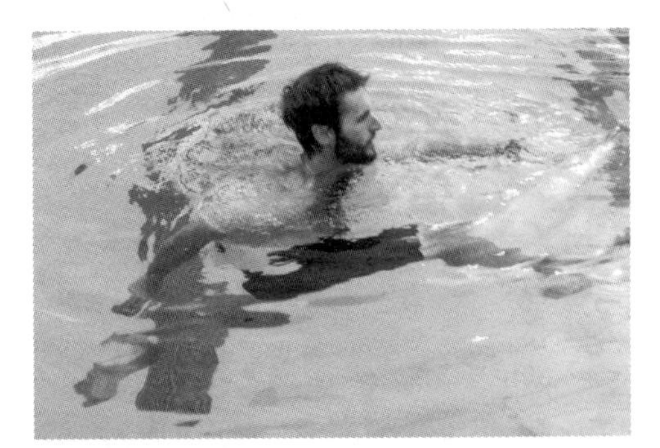

The Cross-Country motion is an opposing swing of the legs straight forward and back.

When performing the Cross-Country, the limbs are strongly grounded in the abdominals in order to support the increased power and to stabilize the lower back/ spine. Begin with legs held with a slight bend (this keeps the hips "unlocked") and the feet in slight dorsiflexion, ankles held softly, not locked. The motion of the Cross-Country is an opposing swing of the legs straight forward and back, maintaining the slight knee bend and relaxed or dorsiflexed foot. When performing the Cross-Country leg motion, think of it like a repetitive soccer kick. The participant should only move the legs in a comfortable range of motion; don't over- or under-reach. Keep the stroke balanced—the reach in front should be equal to the reach to the rear. The Cross-Country, when performed correctly, will increase ROM of the hips due to a stretching effect as the moving limbs (more so the legs) encounter resistance in the water.

While the legs are moving, swing the arms and legs opposite from each other to counter the motion with the opposing limb; personal trainer Douglas Brooks calls this creating "simultaneous stabilization." Coordinating the arms and legs can be challenging for deep water novices, so you can initially do the movement with the leg motion only (with hands on hips). Once mastered, incorporate the upper-body motion.

To perform the upper-body motion with an Open Hand, extend one arm forward, palm facing down and just below the surface of the water. That's the start of the stroke. Keep your head looking forward as the arm powers through the water. When the hand passes your hips, slightly rotate your palm inward toward your body, almost grazing your body with your palm. As the arm continues to move back, the palm will rotate the other way so the thumb ends up pointing away from the body (palm facing down), 8 to 10 inches below the surface of the water.

This swing will rotate the torso slightly and externally (outward) rotate the shoulder when the arm extends back. Think of it as if you were trying to grab something (say, a water bottle) in the back seat of your car without looking back, keeping your head pointed forward at all times. In order to grab the bottle, the arm has to rotate at the shoulder to increase the reach and grip the object. If not, you're attempting to pick up the bottle with the back of your hand. This is very important—without the rotation and the correct palm position, the power through the core cannot be achieved.

I introduce the Cross-Country as a traveling forward stroke before I teach the stationary version because it's easier for participants to develop proper technique and learn the stroke mechanics. It's also more natural to travel through the water than to stay in one place. Make sure you master the movement patterns and overall stroke of the traveling version before trying the stationary one.

To travel forward, the power phase of the stroke needs to occur when the limbs move from the forward position to the back position. To travel backward, reverse the power phase of the stroke to starting in the back position and moving forward.

To master the stationary Cross-Country, you need to create a perfect balance of power by pulling your upper and lower limbs equally; from front to back and back to front. It may take more than one session for a participant to master the full power of the non-traveling Cross-Country.

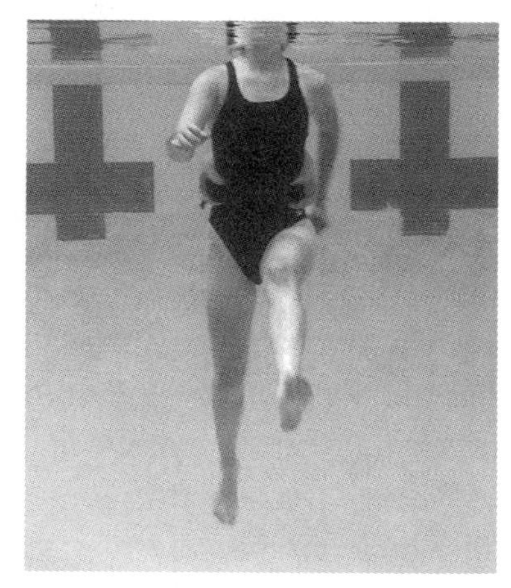

Demonstrating the Closed Hand Cross Country.

The shoulder and hand rotation and reach facilitates an increased range of motion through the torso and will allow the body to produce an intense power phase when the arm returns to the start position. This is one of the keys to the stationary Cross-Country. Recognize that both arms are swinging opposite each other, pulling equally as strong from the front to the back as with the back to the front to keep the body from moving forward.

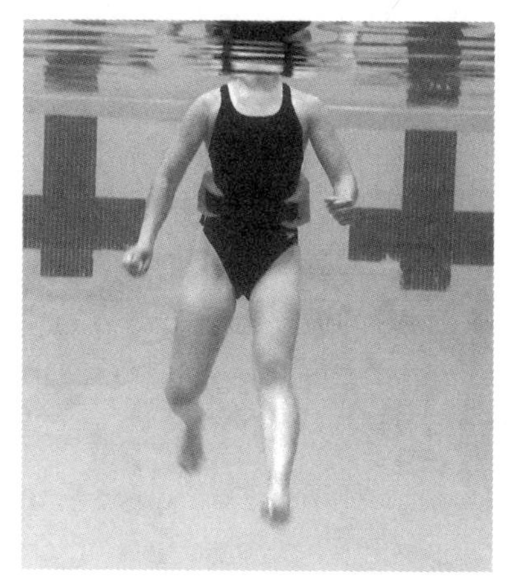

Incorrect with leg width too far apart.

If trying hand position variations, the arm should still swing through the water exactly in the same manner as described using an Open Hand (see page 31). I find utilizing the Slicing Hand awkward with the Cross-Country (especially when the hand/arm is rotating in the back position) so I tend not to use this hand position option.

FORM ISSUES

Unequal power, type 1. For the Stationary (non-traveling) Cross-Country. When more power is delivered from the backward or forward phase of the stroke, you can travel. To correct, perform the Cross-Country with the legs only and hands on the hips. To equalize the power and remain stationary, power harder in the weaker direction. For example, if traveling forward, use more power when the limb is moving from the back position to the forward position and vice versa.

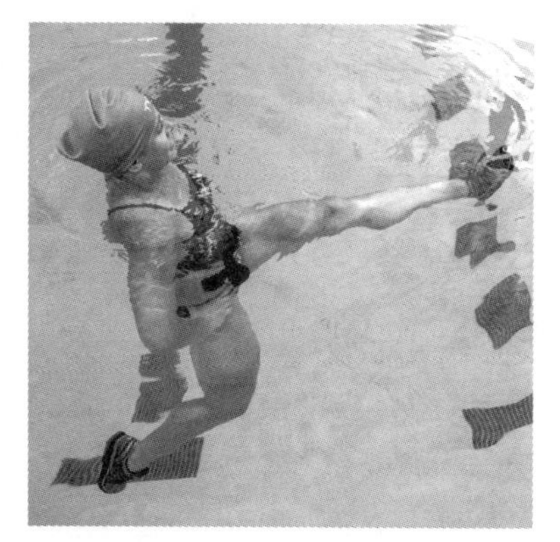

Incorrect leg swing, no rear reach; upper body in correct position.

Unequal power, type 2. When you produce more power with either an upper or lower limb, it appears as an unsynchronized movement or a limp. To balance this unequal power, isolate the stroke by using only the legs or only the arms. By doing so, you'll focus on one part of the body (upper/lower) and isolate the motion. Stay in one place (i.e., non-traveling). For legs only, perform the motions with your hands on your hips and practice the method in Type 1. For arms only, hold the legs straight down; they can be crossed at the ankles or held slightly apart, too. Don't overreach the arms, especially in the back position, and focus on the core to stabilize the stroke. The arms-only version is a highly skilled motion that requires adequate upper-body strength and shoulder joint stability; it's much more difficult for deconditioned or new deep water participants.

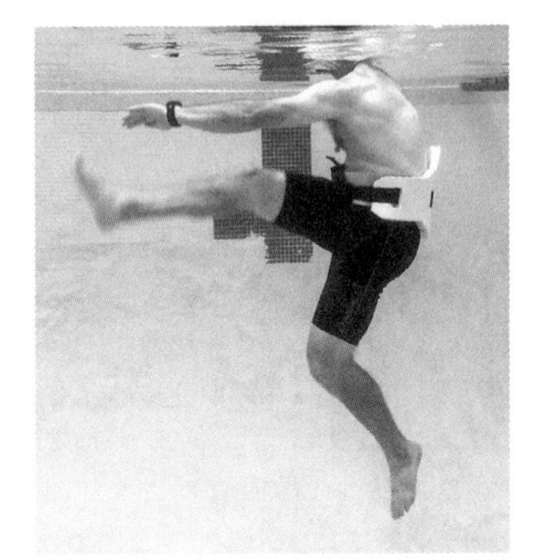

Incorrect excessive forward leg reach with no backward reach of arms or legs.

Locked knees. When knees are locked straight, a chain reaction occurs with the lower body, limiting the hip ROM and shortening the leg stroke. This makes the movement overly robotic and the fluid nature of the stroke disappears. The locked hips force the core to disengage, and the power is then generated only by the limbs. To correct this, relax the knees and keep them slightly bent.

Hitched shoulders. This is when the shoulders ride upward toward the ears in a shrug. To fix, lengthen the spine and keep the shoulders down. If you're aware of it, it can be corrected quite quickly.

Overreaching. Participants may attempt to gain more power by overreaching their legs. This causes the hip/pelvis to shift forward and backward, extending beyond the natural range of motion; it no longer maintains alignment with the spine. The stroke should follow a person's natural range of motion.

Stiff torso/lack of rotation. When the torso doesn't rotate back as the arm is moving behind the body in preparation for the next power phase, the reach is shortened and the power significantly diminished. The telltale sign is when the arm stops around the hip, never achieving a backward reach. Remind participants about slightly rotating the torso when reaching for the "water bottle"; this typically corrects the swing.

PT POINTS

The Cross-Country's increased trunk rotation and intensified power phases can be problematic for those who've had back surgeries or spinal fusion, so pay close attention to abdominal or back pain. The strong power phase (when moving from back to front) in particular requires strong abdominal contraction to stabilize the spine from bending or arching backward.

A locked-out knee puts undue strain on the structures at the knee when powering the leg against the water's resistance. To unlock it, simply bend the knee slightly. But beware: The intense power phases can cause knee strain/pain even if the knee isn't locked out. If you've had knee issues and/or surgery, consult your healthcare team before trying this stroke.

The rotation of the hand facing downward at the end of the back stroke, just before starting the power phase of pulling forward, puts the shoulder in an outwardly rotated and extended position. If you've had shoulder surgery or shoulder dislocation problems, and/or biceps muscle or tendon issues, this position and the action of pulling forward against the water's resistance could be uncomfortable or may not be indicated. Consult with your therapist or physician.

HOW TO INSTRUCT FROM THE DECK

With one leg grounded on the pool deck, perform the same countering arm and leg swing described above, emphasizing the foot dorsiflexion, unlocked knees, and reach back with the arm, palms rotated downward. Demonstrations may involve rotating in place on the pool deck to be sure people can see what's being demonstrated from any angle, especially with specific cues or when emphasizing certain limb positions during the stroke. It's acceptable to even stop and freeze mid-stroke to point out certain aspects, such as the knee or the reach behind the body. Useful terms and phrases include:

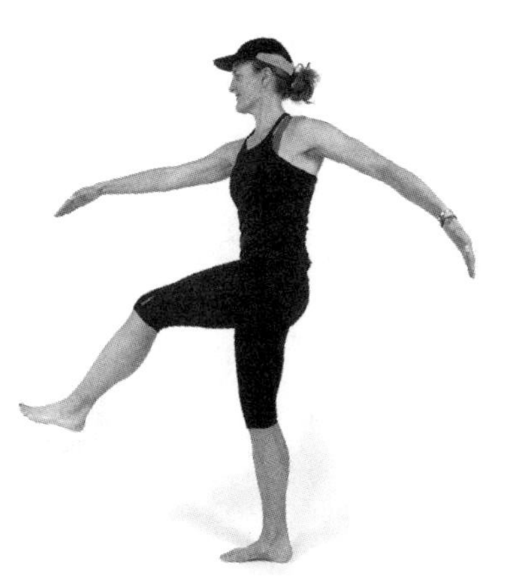

Demonstrating the Cross-Country with an Open Hand.

- *Range of motion first, then power.* This will allow participants to find their rhythm and the range of motion of their arms and legs before increasing their power.
- *Pretend you're grabbing your water bottle from the back seat of your car.* This is to help them remember to keep their heads forward while rotating the shoulder and palm to mimic picking something up while driving.
- *Keep your joints strong yet relaxed. Don't lock out.*
- *Feel your abs/core working.* This will remind participants that their core should stay engaged during the entire driving action forward and backward.
- *It's okay to rotate through your torso.* This is always a good reminder for any stroke that requires a rotation.

HOW TO USE THIS STROKE IN A WORKOUT

In introducing the Cross-Country for the first time, I have a group maintain the stroke for several minutes, pointing out every aspect of the stroke. Then, for the second minute, I have them push hard for 10 seconds and go easy for 10 to get used to the power phase.

HIGH KNEE

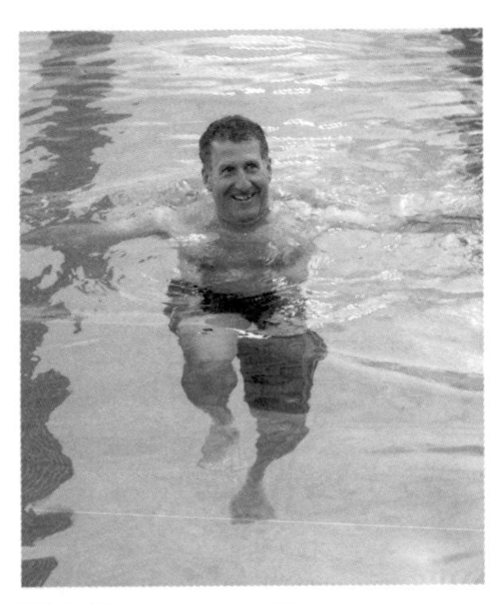

High Knee start position, arms sculling.

Picture a football player running line drills through a single line of tires: feet moving from inside the tire to outside before moving into the next tire, legs pumping up and down—fast and high. Or visualize your knees coming high up to your waist like a soccer player launching a ball up with their knees then driving the leg down toward the ground. Now imagine doing this in the water without touching the floor of the pool and think of the tremendous impact water resistance has on the legs moving at this high speed. The High Knee is intense—so intense that it's used primarily for sprinting efforts, an exercise performed in short bursts of about 15 seconds. Performing this exercise at much longer durations will be difficult as the speed and range of motion of the legs may not be sustained due to muscle fatigue and the high anaerobic nature of the stroke. This difficult stroke leads participants to instinctively seek easier ways to perform it. If you find the High Knee seems easy, I can guarantee you're not performing it correctly.

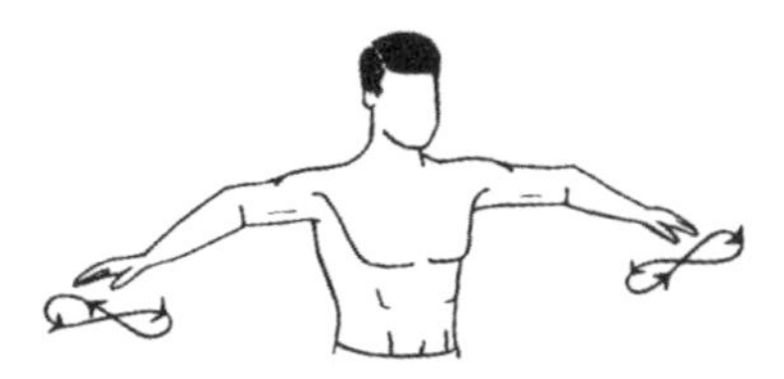

Sculling arm.

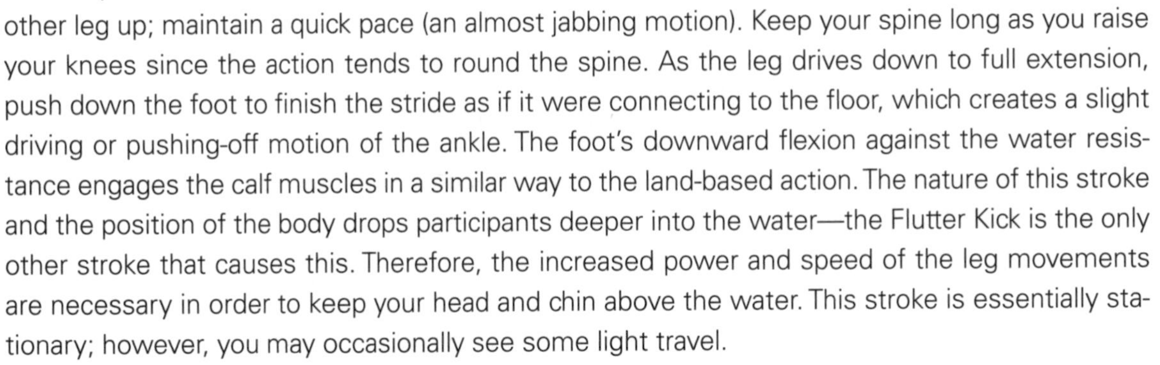

To perform the High Knee, keep your body upright and vertical with no noticeable lean. Start by bringing one knee high toward your chest and then, as you lower the leg, bring the other leg up; maintain a quick pace (an almost jabbing motion). Keep your spine long as you raise your knees since the action tends to round the spine. As the leg drives down to full extension, push down the foot to finish the stride as if it were connecting to the floor, which creates a slight driving or pushing-off motion of the ankle. The foot's downward flexion against the water resistance engages the calf muscles in a similar way to the land-based action. The nature of this stroke and the position of the body drops participants deeper into the water—the Flutter Kick is the only other stroke that causes this. Therefore, the increased power and speed of the leg movements are necessary in order to keep your head and chin above the water. This stroke is essentially stationary; however, you may occasionally see some light travel.

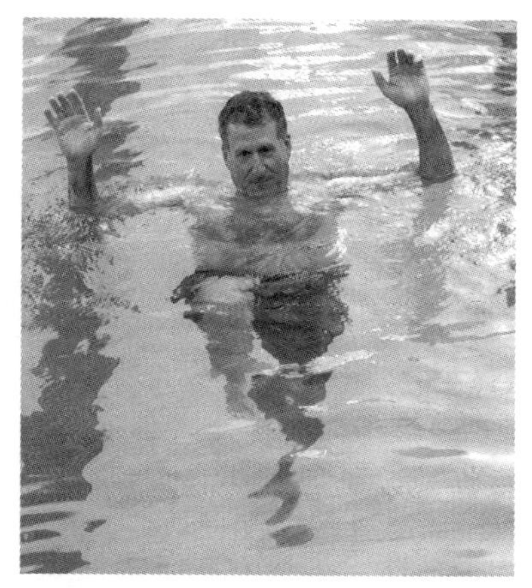
Raise your arms above the water to increase the difficulty of this already intense stroke.

When introducing the High Knee, start with your arms parallel to the water surface, sculling the water. To scull, hold your hands palms down (toward the pool bottom) and make a sweeping figure-eight (or infinity sign) along the plane of the water's surface; the full motion covers about 8 inches of water. Sculling helps keep the head above water and the body higher in the pool with the least amount of effort, which enables you to focus more on body alignment and how the legs should drive through the water. Sculling can be used to both prepare for the start of the stroke as well as used as a recovery.

As mentioned, the High Knee is an intense stroke. To significantly increase its difficulty, raise your arms above the water. The higher your hands are raised out of the water, the more rigorous the exercise becomes as the body sinks deeper in the water. Start the High Knee with the scull then transition to the arms aligned with the sides of the body, elbows at 90 degrees, and chest open; the arms should be outside the peripheral vision. Keeping the elbows out to the sides is more intense compared to the elbows pointed forward, which is another acceptable variation. Those who are gluttons for punishment can raise their arms even higher, which sinks the body farther down and makes the workout even more challenging because the legs must work even harder.

Here are two other variations that can be performed with the High Knee.

1. Lightly touch the lower part of the back of the head. This will make the body actually sink, sometimes up to several inches, forcing an even harder workload than when the arms are simply raised above the head. It's important to continue keeping the chin just at or above the water line, head pointing directly forward.

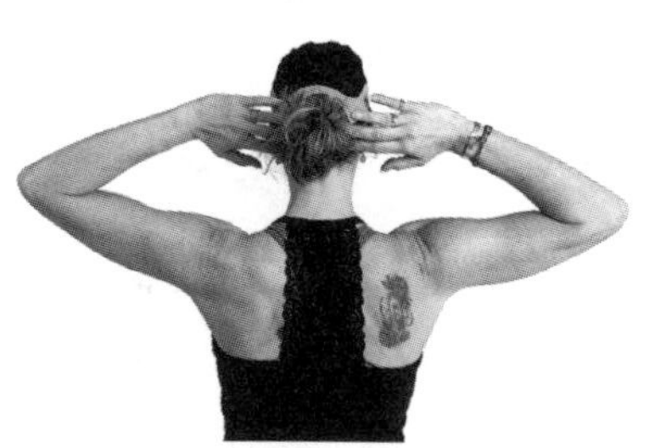
Touching the back of your head while doing the High Knee will force you to work harder to maintain the proper body position.

2. A variation of this stroke is to perform the movement with a wider stance to resemble the football training drill with a ladder of tires, two abreast. This incorporates more abductor/adductor muscles of the hip/leg.

FORM ISSUES

Disengaged core. Typically, participants disengage their core and hitch their hips behind them with a rounded upper back, which creates more buoyancy in their torso. When doing so, the stroke's intensity decreases considerably. Keep a tall spine with hips aligned under the shoulders. A good visual clue is to look down in the water; if you see the tops of your thighs when your legs are driven to the full downward position, then you're hitching your hips back. The thighs aren't visible when using proper form.

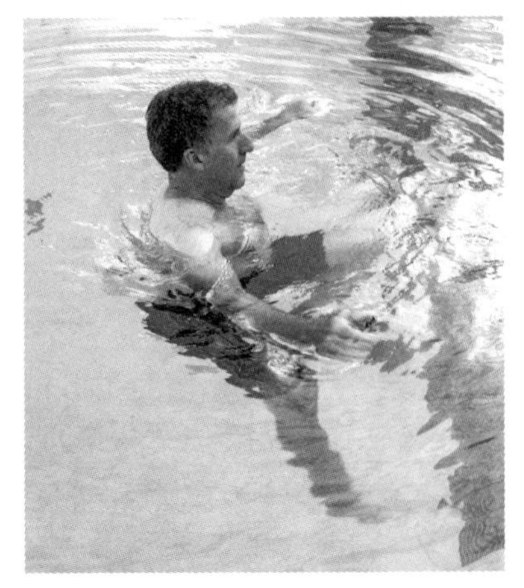

Incorrect: legs and arms too far forward.

Eggbeating legs. If you come from a synchronized swimming or water polo background, you tend to "eggbeat" your legs, which works well for your sport. This type of continuous circular motion is actually easier to perform than the High Knee as it keeps your head higher above the water with less effort. To correct, attempt to "step on a spot" just underneath you to keep your legs moving vertically up and down.

Poor body/neck alignment. When you try to work harder, your head may tilt back so that your face looks straight up. This compromises your neck and your entire body alignment. Remember, keep a tall spine with your hips under your shoulders and your face pointed forward.

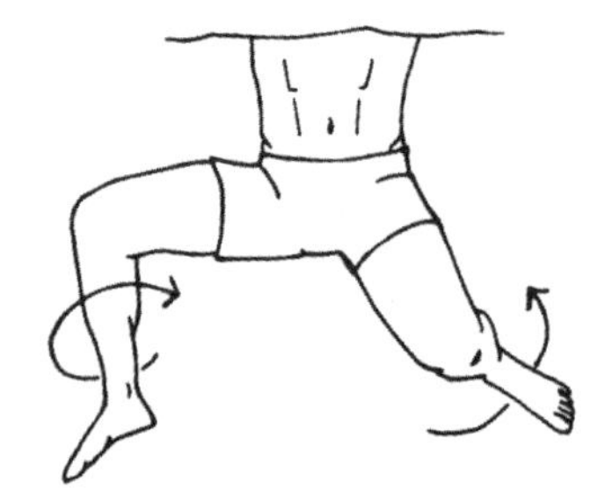

Don't eggbeat your legs—this makes the stroke easier.

PT POINTS

With the legs pumping up and down so quickly and forcefully, solid core stability is crucial. This exercise isn't recommended for those still recovering from lower limb, abdominal, or spine surgery and/or injury until sufficient strength and conditioning has been regained.

If the neck is flexed backward, it can exert excessive pressure on the soft tissues and bony components of the neck, which can create a variety of problems, including but not limited to pain and dizziness. Correct this form error immediately especially if there has been any prior neck surgery or injury.

Also, don't shrug the shoulders upward. Not only can this cause neck discomfort and strain, it will limit arm motion during sculling.

HOW TO INSTRUCT FROM THE DECK

Make sure participants perform the High Knee with proper form—spine elongated, faces forward, and arms sculling at the sides. You can demonstrate this quite easily even using both legs, marching on the deck of the pool. Then have participants slowly raise their arms above the water while still maintaining proper body position. The higher the arms are raised out of the water, the farther the body drops into the water, so the legs will need to work at a hard and quick pace for the body to maintain proper form (i.e., tall spine, head/chin above water, face looking forward). Allow participants to first "test out" the motion, especially with the arms raised, to get themselves used to the sensation of sinking down several inches, and then experiment with maintaining proper body position without using the arms for stability and balance. This is also another opportunity to verbally assist with adjustments. Useful terms and phrases include:

- *Keep your body upright.* This helps them keep proper body alignment.
- *Drive down through the stroke.* This keeps the leg driving through as if planting on the floor, as typically the leg will stop short of a full leg extension.
- *Elbows out, head forward.* This helps with proper full-body alignment when working at threshold/high efforts.

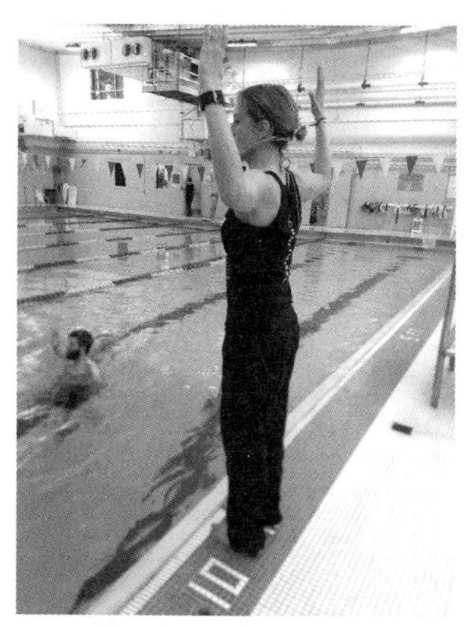

Demonstrating the arms at a 90-degree.

HOW TO USE THIS STROKE IN A WORKOUT

When the arms are above the water, the High Knee is an intense interval exercise so this works well when the fitness goal is to work a participant at 85% effort (or above) during interval training. Try the High Knee in a set of 15 seconds at 85%, then take a break for 15 (repeat three or four times).

FLUTTER KICK

The Flutter Kick works well in a workout set that alternates with the High Knee because both have a similar stationary position and upright body alignment. The body is held vertically in the water, legs hanging straight down below the individual with relaxed knees (not locked out) and feet typically pointed downward. With a slight knee bend and alternating legs, kick forward and backward rapidly (approximately 10 to 12 inches) to attempt to drive the body up and out of the water. This is a similar motion used to propel across the pool with a kickboard or through the water when scuba diving. The powerful quadriceps, hamstrings, and glute muscles come into play here.

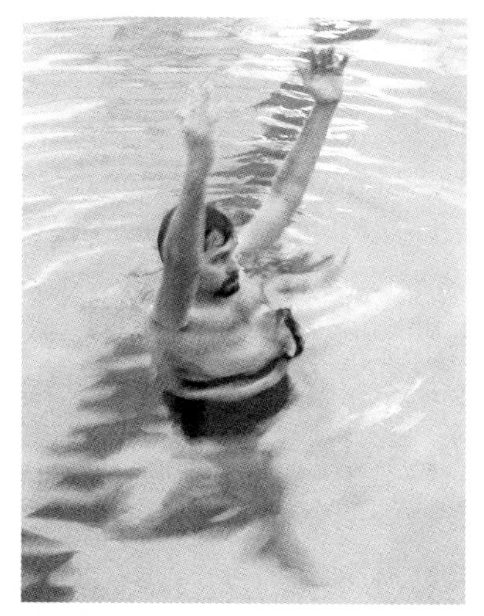

Flutter Kick with raised arms.

When introducing the Flutter Kick, start with sculling, the sweeping motion that traces an infinity sign (or the number eight) along the plane of the water's surface with your arms held straight out at your sides and palms facing the bottom of the pool. Sculling helps keep your body higher in the pool and your head above water with the least amount of effort. Then slowly raise your arms above the water; the higher your arms are held out of the water, the more your body will sink. A greater effort will be needed to keep your chin above water while maintaining proper form. The arm position is the same as the High Knee—arms outside the peripheral vision. To make the move even harder, touch the back of your head, which sinks the body farther down.

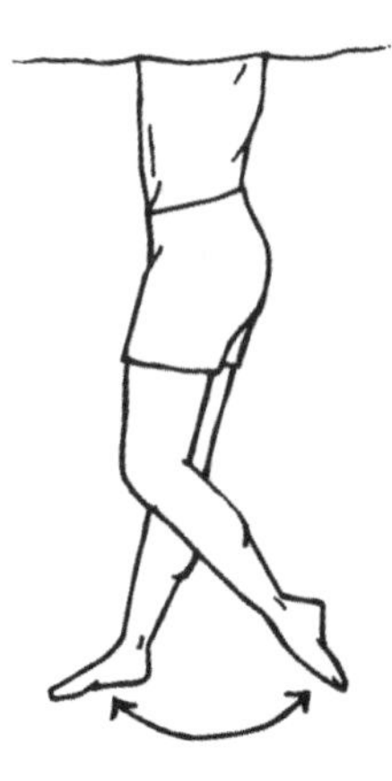

With a slight knee bend and alternating legs, kick forward and backward rapidly.

FORM ISSUES

Locked Hips. A typical issue is kicking from the knees instead of the hips. This happens when the hips are locked to ground the stroke rather than grounding with the core, which allows movement through the hip joints. The primary issue in this case is the difficulty participants have in effectively driving the force of the Flutter Kick from the upper legs down through to the lower leg. Without using the core to ground the stroke, this full-leg motion is difficult to perform correctly. Don't lock the hips; relaxed hips naturally promote more upper leg motion.

PT POINTS

This stroke can be stressful on the knees due to the rapid and forceful movement against the water's resistance, especially if the hips are locked. Decrease the effort level if you experience pain, especially on the front side of your knee. If you have had knee surgery, be cautious with high intensity levels.

HOW TO INSTRUCT FROM THE DECK

This stroke can be demonstrated with one foot on the ground and the other leg hanging over the edge of the pool to show the length and how the leg will swing and kick through the water. This will also allow you to demonstrate the upper body, and point to the muscles in the core, quads, hamstrings, and glutes. Useful terms and phrases include:

- *Keep your body upright.* This helps keep proper body alignment.
- *Drive down through the legs.* This keeps the legs driving through the larger muscles of the upper legs, rather than just the lower legs.
- *Elbows out, hands up, head forward.* This maintains proper form and prevents tilting the head backward.

HOW TO USE THIS STROKE IN A WORKOUT

As with the High Knee, the Flutter Kick is excellent to use for short interval sets. I often pair both strokes together one after another, with recoveries, and sprinkle sets of them throughout a 60-minute workout.

CHAPTER 5

Let's Crank This Up: Advanced Exercises

> *"Studies suggest that adding deep water running to an athlete's training regimen has the potential to increase fitness and ultimately improve performance...it may also be necessary to use an intensity that is similar to that used during land-based training in order for aquatic modalities to be effective."*[43]

Now that you have the foundational hand positions and strokes, you're definitely ready for some advanced strokes. An advanced stroke is not just intense, it's also quite complex. If you're new to hydro exercising, make sure you can do the basics in Chapter 4 before you begin learning these more complicated movements.

As with the strokes in Chapter 4, each description includes the focused power phase in order to show when and where the power is initiated. The power is sometimes balanced between both the backward and forward motions. It can also come from one direction, with a recovery phase for the opposite motion. The descriptions don't usually contain specifics of the recovery phase as each individual will discover a pattern of recovery that works for them. When recovery is mentioned, however, there's an important aspect that needs to be addressed.

Due to differences with individual ROM, flexibility, and muscular strength, remember that the limb movement, torso rotation, and start/finish positions of participants may vary. Despite these differences, it's important to maintain proper form.

For safety reasons, all demonstrations by a coach/trainer should be made with one foot planted on the pool deck. This position requires good balance, so if additional support is needed (such as a chair, rail, or other equipment for balance assistance), plan ahead.

WATER WALK

The Water Walk takes the Water Run motion and adds a twist to the torso and an extension of the limbs to create a sweeping power stroke that will make a person travel through the water. Water Walking is performed as if attempting to wipe your arm across a table in an outward sweeping motion while doing the same type of broad sweeping stroke with the opposite leg. I also refer to this move as a speed skater on the moon (not that I actually know what that's like). These are larger-than-normal strides/strokes because they sweep back and away from the midline of the body. The recovery of this stroke involves bringing the limbs back to the start position in a natural path that glides the feet and hands back to the start position with the least amount of water resistance. When performed by experienced individuals, it looks so easy and graceful that it isn't perceived as difficult.

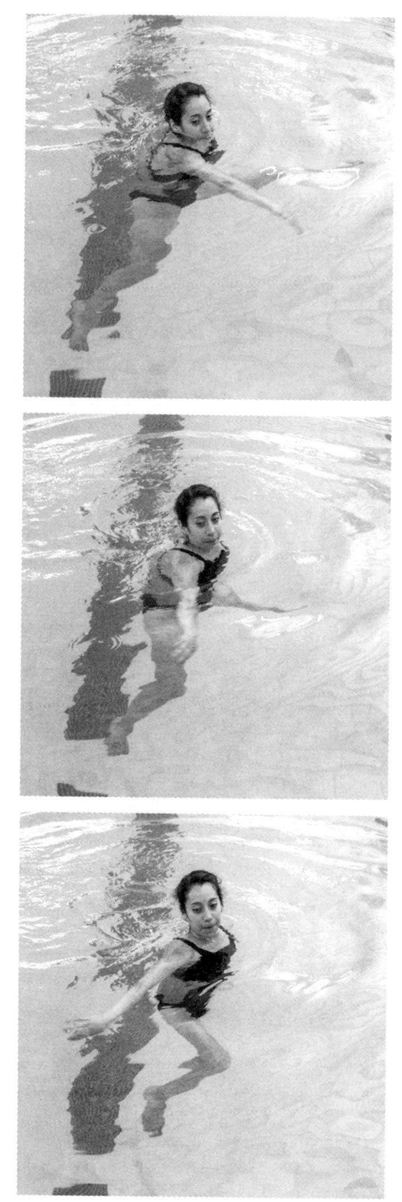

From top to bottom: start, pull and follow-through of Water Walk.

To get to the start of the upper-body power phase, extend your right (starting) arm straight out in front of your body several inches below the surface of the water, just crossing over the midline to your left side. Your elbow should be almost straight. This is where the power begins. Now sweep your arm back and to the right at a slight downward angle, to the back position, finishing with your arm slightly behind your body, 10 to 12 inches under water. Engagement of the upper back and scapular muscles also opens the chest area. Your shoulders shouldn't roll forward or shrug up toward your ears. This motion naturally incorporates a trunk rotation with the forward reach followed by a smooth, powerful stroke to the end position.

Now let's define the power phase of the lower body with the corresponding left (starting) leg. The leg starts in front, close to the midline of the body or even crossing over slightly to the right. Drive your leg through the water with an outward sweeping motion. The leg motion differs from person to person depending on flexibility and range of motion.

In its perfected form, this stroke uses a wide range of motion of the hip and shoulder joints. The core strength required to ground the forces generated in this stroke is much greater because of the increased trunk rotation and the lever arm that's created by the limbs traveling farther away from the body.

FORM ISSUES

Lack of core engagement and stability. The stroke will look choppy instead of smooth when you don't engage the core sufficiently. This is one of the hardest issues to correct. As an instructor, demonstrate the lack of core involvement by swinging the limbs quickly, with a relaxed or loose core, and point at your abdominal area to emphasize this point (yes, more participant laughter).

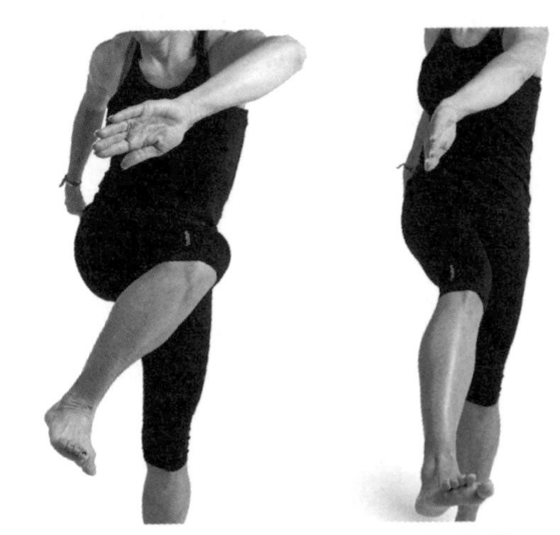

Don't hike your hip during the stroke (left). To correct, lower the leg and extend the knee (right).

Hip hike. It's common for someone with limited flexibility or in the learning stages to hike up the hip and pelvis when trying to lift the leg higher and bring it closer to midline. This actually rolls the entire leg inward, bringing the knee closer to the midline instead of the foot. With the hip hiked and leg starting in this position for the power stroke, the hip joint will lose its ability to sweep to the side and fully extend backward and the knee will remain flexed, all of which prevent the leg from generating power. To correct the hike, lower the leg and extend the knee. This will encourage joint movement within one's natural range.

PT POINTS

This exercise isn't appropriate for those who've had posterior/lateral-approach hip replacement/arthroplasty and/or a hip dislocation, and haven't yet been cleared for full activity and full range of motion without any precautions. This is because of the leg's starting point: crossed over the midline, flexed at the hip, and potentially inwardly rotated. These positions don't comply with the standard posterior/lateral-approach hip-replacement precautions.

Additionally, shoulder hitching/shrugging, especially with the wide sweeping motion of the arm, can lead to compression or impingement of the shoulder joint. If you have shoulder impingement issues, take note of your shoulder position and assess for pain during the power phase of this stroke. Adjust as needed.

HOW TO INSTRUCT FROM THE DECK

Moving slowly while demonstrating is critical to show the distinctions of this stroke. Start with a motion that's very similar to that slow-moving speed skater on the moon, mentioned earlier. Swing the right leg forward, leading with the heel. At near full extension in front, create a slight scooping action with the foot and then sweep back in an outward arch to a point slightly behind your body. At the same time, the opposing arm should be moving at the same pace and sweep as described in the main description, as if you were trying to wipe a table off with your arm all in one motion. Useful terms and phrases regarding the reach and the drive needed in the Water Walk include:

- The range of motion should feel natural and flowing.
- Allow the lower body to move naturally.
- Follow-through on the stroke.
- Feel your lower and your upper body counter each other.
- Core and form before power.
- This is a powerful and smooth stroke.

HOW TO USE THIS STROKE IN A WORKOUT

The Water Walk is one of my favorite strokes for a warm-up or a recovery, but I also use it for a steady-state effort or a hard interval set typically lasting 1 to 2 minutes.

REVERSE WATER WALK

The Reverse Water Walk is one of two exercises that uses the Reverse Hand (page 35). Using the same Water Walk arm motion, rotate the arm so that the thumb points up but with the arm still under the surface of the water. The arm will move in a similar outward sweeping motion but lead with the back of the hand. Another difference is that the arm finishes slightly lower in the water to further promote upper back engagement and scapula retraction, which is the focus on this variation. There will be some traveling, but not at the same speed as with the regular hand position. By promoting the upper/mid-back (i.e., scapular muscles, the posterior shoulder muscles, and increased involvement of the latissimus dorsi), this change in the hand position lessens the involvement of the upper deltoid and upper shoulder region. The Reverse Hand stroke, which targets these muscle groups, is highly beneficial for a range of individuals from desk jockeys to distance cyclists. Both spend inordinate amounts of time hunched forward in a turtle posture and therefore have weak, stretched upper back muscles and tight chests.

FORM ISSUES

Locked wrist. The Reverse Hand position is prone to locked wrists, which leads one to power the arm stroke with primarily the wrist/forearm instead of engaging the back and shoulders. This seemingly minor issue of a locked wrist can create intense tension through the forearm (see PT Points below). Rather than leading with the wrist, drive through the stroke by first engaging the larger muscle groups of the upper back and shoulder.

Raised/shrugged shoulders. Raised or shrugged shoulders cause participants to pull their arms through the water much higher and closer to the surface than they should be. This position will drive the stroke with the deltoids rather than the back/scapular muscles, making the sweeping motion look choppy instead of smooth. To correct this issue, drive the arm downward so that it finishes 10 to 12 inches underwater.

PT POINTS

In the Reverse Hand position, increased pressure is put at the wrist joint to stabilize the wrist against the force of the water. Attention must be given to pain and/or fatigue in these muscles controlling the wrist. Refer to the expanded explanation in the Reverse Hand PT Points (page 35).

The other important consideration with this stroke is the shoulder motion. As the arms sweep back, the shoulder joint externally rotates (rotates outward). This motion uses the smaller, less-developed muscles along the back side of the shoulder joint, which are part of the rotator cuff. If you've had any type of shoulder surgery or major injury and haven't been cleared for all activity, it's recommended that you discuss this exercise with your therapist and/or physician, specifying this particular hand position and arm motion.

If external shoulder rotation is what you want to strengthen for general balance, function, and stability of the shoulder joint (and you don't fall into the category previously outlined), then this exercise would be very beneficial when executed correctly.

HOW TO INSTRUCT FROM THE DECK

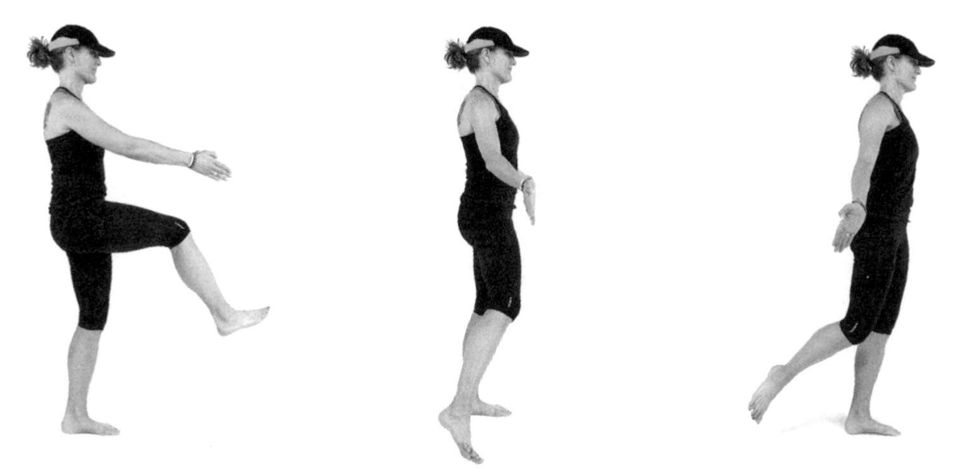

Left to right: start, follow-through, and finish of Reverse Water Walk.

Just as with the Water Walk, demonstrate the entire full-body stroke in slow motion. Then isolate just the arm and Open Hand position, followed by a transition to a Reverse Hand position. This allows the participants to focus on the one element that's changing. Explain that this stroke should be felt in the upper back and between the shoulder blades. Consider pointing to the region to help them identify the location. Useful terms and phrases include:

- Keep the wrist somewhat relaxed.
- Pull through the upper back, not just the shoulder.
- Light torso rotation is okay. This will help engage the core and back.

HOW TO USE THIS STROKE IN A WORKOUT

I like using the Reverse Water Walk for 45 seconds to a minute in between intense quicker strokes like the High Knee and Water Run.

BREAST STROKE

The Breast Stroke isn't easy. However, when performed well, it may look that way! This stroke has some similarities to the Water Walk with the outward sweeping limb movement, except the Breast Stroke powers the arms and legs at the exact same time. All four limbs move away from each other then back in a sweeping motion together at the same time, in contrast to the movement in the Water Walk, Water Run, and the Cross-Country, where the opposite arm and leg move in conjunction with each other.

The upper-body power phase begins with both arms reaching straight out in front of the body, about 6 to 10 inches on either side of the midline, several inches below the surface of the water. The arms power through the water with a forward and downward sweep. They finish at the sides (frontal plane) and transition into the recovery phase approximately at hip level. This stroke engages the upper back and scapular muscles as well as opens the chest. Due to the simultaneous arm strokes, there's no trunk rotation.

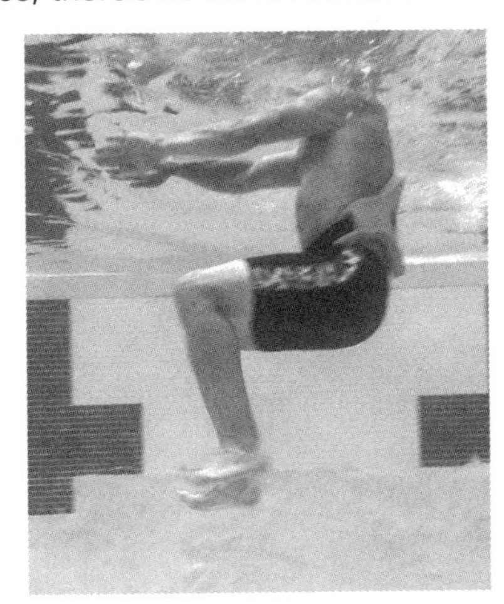

Start

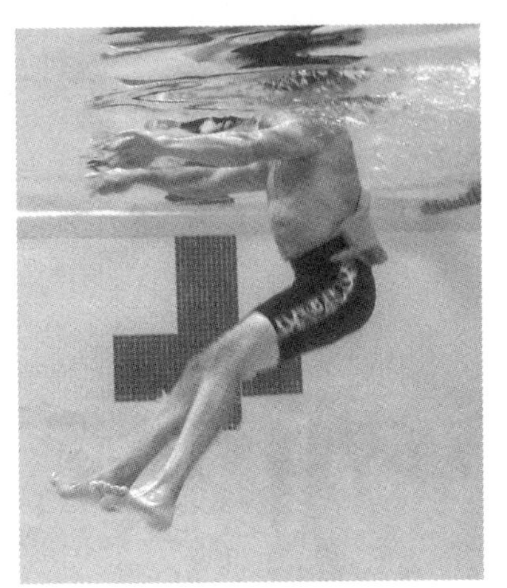

Pull

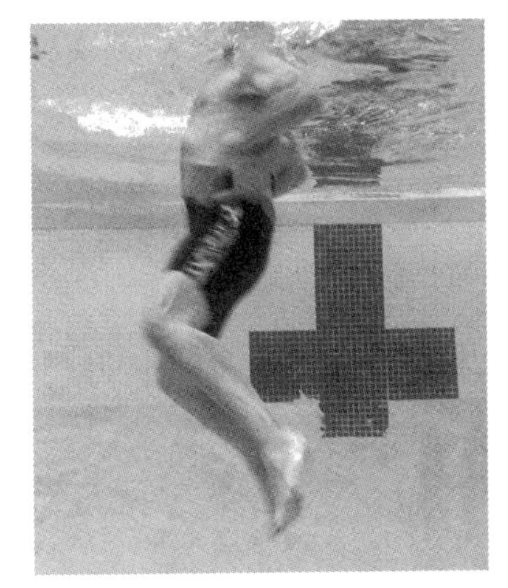

Follow-through

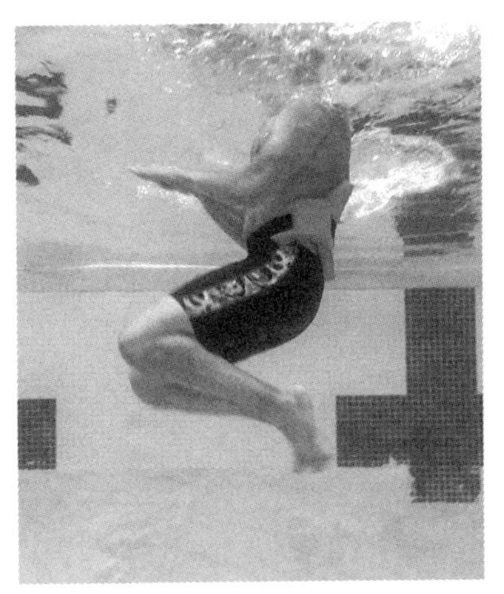

Recovery

For the lower-limb power phase, the starting leg position begins about a foot out on either side of the midline of the body (with your rear almost appearing to be "sitting on a stool") and then pull the legs through with power in an outward sweeping motion. The hips drive forward, with the glutes engaged simultaneously as the legs sweep behind. By leading with the heel and maintaining a knee bend, the stroke finishes with the heel moving up toward the buttock. The lower abs and hip extensors (hamstring/glutes) engage to assist with stabilizing the pelvis, appearing almost as a slow butt tuck.

Take your time and be patient with learning this stroke. I've found that this is by far the hardest stroke to master.

FORM ISSUES

Thrusting the pelvis forward. The main reason for pushing the pelvis forward is a rushed leg motion that doesn't sweep or extend the legs. Often the knee is locked into one position. To correct, extend the legs and pull through the water with the heels, allowing some motion at the knee joint.

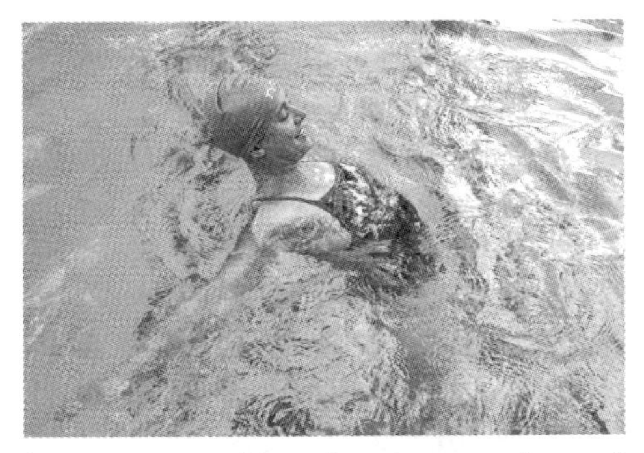

Incorrect excessive and unnecessary forward pelvis thrust.

Upper-body dominance. Your upper body dominates the stroke when you derive most of the power from your shoulders; your arms are high in the water, moving in smaller circles of motion in front and to the sides. To adjust your form, keep your chest forward and sweep your arms in a longer path downward in the water.

PT POINTS

Refer to Water Walk for upper-body PT Points (page 56). Pelvic thrusting can create more motion than is intended at the lower spine, leading to hyperextension of the lower back. Watch for lower back pain and discomfort. Be sure to engage the core and tighten the gluteals.

HOW TO INSTRUCT FROM THE DECK

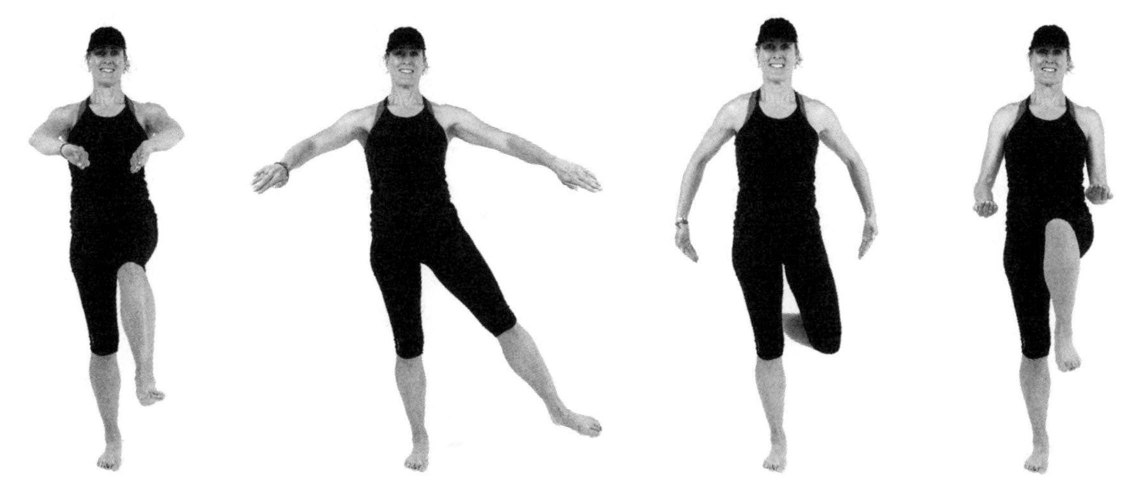

From left to right: demonstrating the Breast Stroke's start, pull-through, finish, and recovery.

The Breast Stroke is one of the more difficult strokes to instruct from the deck. Plant one foot on the deck and slowly move through the motions with one leg and both arms. Keep in mind that emphasizing the arm motion, where the hand finishes, and the goal to drive through the pelvis without thrusting are key to learning this stroke. Yet again, this is a demonstration that could produce chuckles. I refer to it as my "Tom Jones" hips (yes, I just dated myself). To help engage the muscles at the finish of the stroke rather than quickly shifting to recovery, I have participants isometrically hold the pulled-back position, glutes and the mid-back/scapular region tightened for 1 second before the recovery phase (I call it "hang time"). Useful terms and phrases include:

- Drive smoothly through the stroke, careful not to thrust the pelvis.
- Feel your core, hamstrings, and glutes.
- Try not to rush the stroke. Hang time a bit.

HOW TO USE THIS STROKE IN A WORKOUT

I recommend using the Breast Stroke in sets from 30 seconds up to several minutes at a time, depending on the intensity desired.

LEGS-ONLY BREAST STROKE/ARMS-ONLY BREAST STROKE

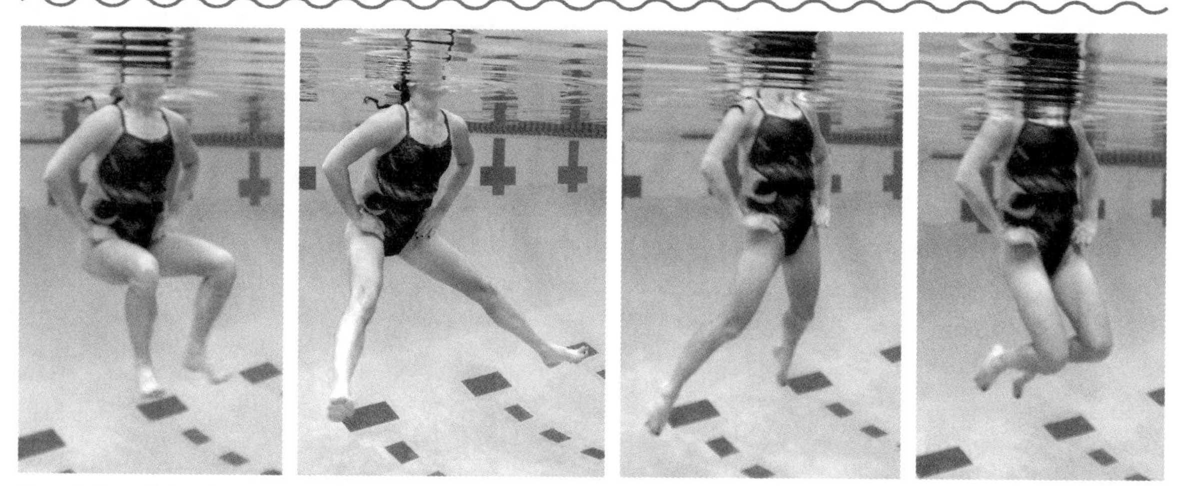

From left to right: the Legs-Only Breast Stroke's start, pull, follow-through, and recovery.

When someone is struggling to master the simultaneous leg and arm motions during the learning process, I use the Legs-Only or Arms-Only Breast Stroke in order to focus on just one part of the body at a time. This method can also be used for targeted strengthening of either the upper or lower body.

Start with isolating the lower body, which provides the momentum and establishes the proper posture in the water. To start the Breast Stroke Legs-Only, place your hands on your hips. This isolates the leg motion and allows you to focus on proper leg position and motion as well as how to best generate power.

However, I don't recommend starting immediately with an Arms-Only Breast Stroke. You won't have enough momentum to secure the upright body position when starting the stroke without the use of the legs. This leads to too much strain on the shoulders. So begin by doing both the leg and arm movements; once you gain enough momentum from your lower body to stay upright, slowly stop using your legs. To do so, relax your legs; you can also cross the ankles and hold them in a relaxed position. As this happens, focus on the arms, particularly the sweep and downward stroke. Perform three to five strokes with arms only, then have the legs rejoin the movement; repeat as needed. Limit the number of consecutive arms-only strokes to maintain good upper-body form.

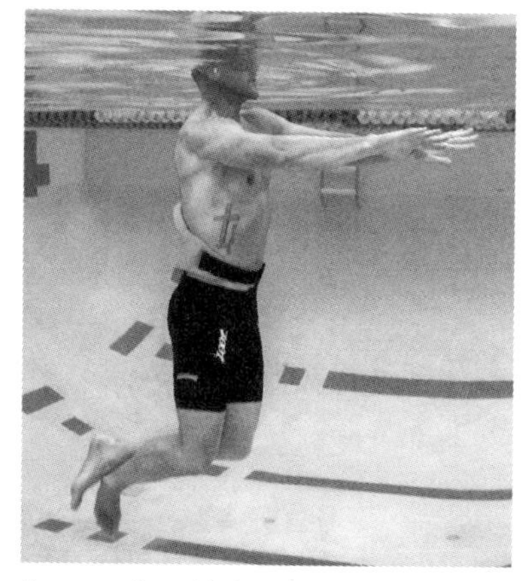
Arms only with knees bent.

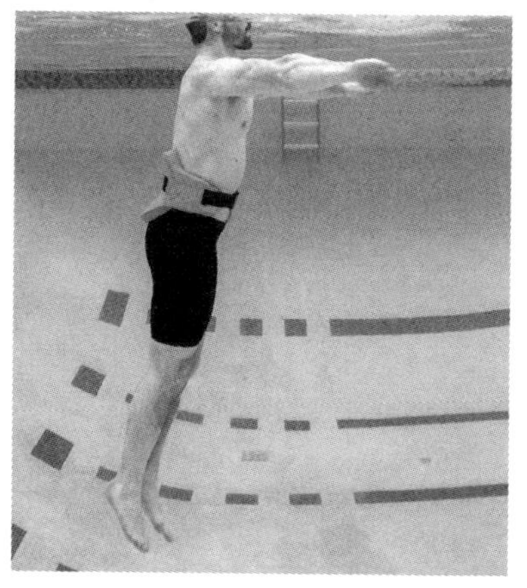
Arms only with legs straight.

FORM ISSUES

An Arms-Only Breast Stroke is quite strenuous on the upper body and can provoke muscle/joint discomfort or strain if used by individuals who have weak shoulders or past/current injuries. (See Breast Stroke PT Points on page 61.)

PT POINTS

With the Arms-Only Breast Stroke, the power phase requires significantly more strength and stability of the shoulder, upper body, and the entire core because there are no countering forces of the legs. Master the Legs-Only stroke first to develop conditioning and stability of the core, and familiarize yourself with how this stroke feels. By doing this, you'll have a more solid foundation to anchor the strenuous Arms-Only stroke. Watch for shoulder strain/pain and adjust accordingly. It's possible that this stroke is simply too taxing for some to perform comfortably or safely. (See Breast Stroke PT Points on page 61.)

HOW TO INSTRUCT FROM THE DECK

See the Breast Stroke notes on page 61.

HOW TO USE THIS STROKE IN A WORKOUT

The legs-only or arms-only versions are perfect to use in a workout set to learn and/or correct form or to work within an interval to increase the intensity. Have participants work within a set that provides a series of these three Breast Stroke variations: the standard, the Legs-Only and the Arms-Only.

REVERSE BREAST STROKE

Once you've mastered the Breast Stroke, try it with a Reverse Hand position. The purpose of this stroke is to isolate and focus on the upper back muscles, as described in Reverse Water Walk (page 57).

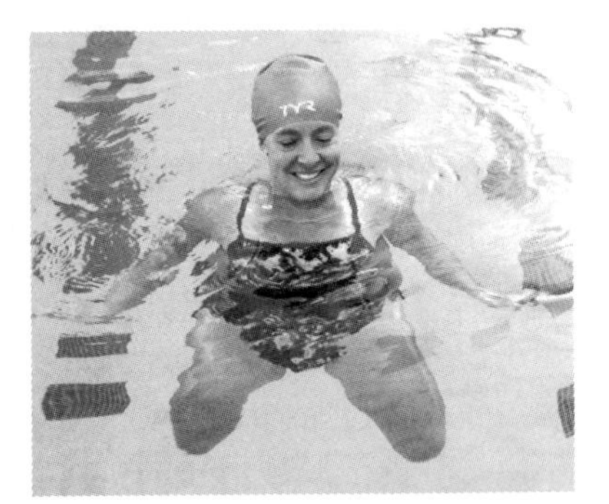

The Reverse Breast Stroke focuses on the upper back muscles.

The starting arm position and motion is very different from the regular Breast Stroke. To begin, rotate the arm so that the thumb points up. Then extend the arms out in front only about half the distance away from the body of the Breast Stroke starting position and 6 to 10 inches below the surface of the water. The arms are held bent at the elbows with the elbows somewhat close to the sides of the body. The power begins when you initiate a backward sweep, leading with the back of the hand, moving from the midline to the frontal plane (external rotation of the shoulder). The elbows don't travel away from the body as with the Breast Stroke; rather, they remain close to the body at almost waist level. Because the arm is bent, you'll feel less drag/resistance, leading to a potentially higher turnover than the Breast Stroke. Even with a higher arm cadence, the shorter reach may slow the travel speed compared to the standard Breast Stroke.

The legs move the same way as in the Breast Stroke but faster to match the quicker upper-body cadence.

FORM ISSUES

Overreaching arm. At any point in the stroke, if you overreach your arms, your elbows will drift outward and away from your body, which compromises your form. This extended arm position diminishes the full strengthening benefits to the upper back and causes excessive tension in the shoulders. To correct, keep your elbows down and closer to your body. You'll feel this stroke in your upper back and between your shoulder blades.

PT POINTS

This advanced stroke requires more power production through the arm stroke, especially from the smaller muscle groups of the shoulder. Please see the Reverse Hand PT Points (page 35) for wrist and elbow concerns, and the Reverse Water Walk PT Points (page 58) for the shoulders. If you've had any type of shoulder surgery or major injury and haven't been cleared for all activity, it's recommended that you clear this exercise with your therapist and/or physician, specifying this particular hand position and arm motion.

HOW TO INSTRUCT FROM THE DECK

See Breast Stroke's How to Instruct from the Deck on page 61. However, during the demonstration, keep elbows down closer your waist as described above.

HOW TO USE THIS STROKE IN A WORKOUT

Use the Reverse Breast Stroke to break up regular Breast Stroke for increased isolation of the upper back muscles. It's a great stroke for mid-length drills of 30 seconds to even a minute.

CROSS-COUNTRY POP-UP

This stroke begins with the Cross-Country motion you already learned on page 43; however, the power phase of the Pop-Up changes to only the part of the stroke where the limbs are pulled toward the body (one half of the full stroke). The recovery phase then becomes the part of the stroke where the limbs are moving away from the body. The power phase propels the body straight up and out of the water by several inches in some cases, higher out of the water than a standard Cross-Country. This engages the core more for stability, with the greater power generated by the limbs.

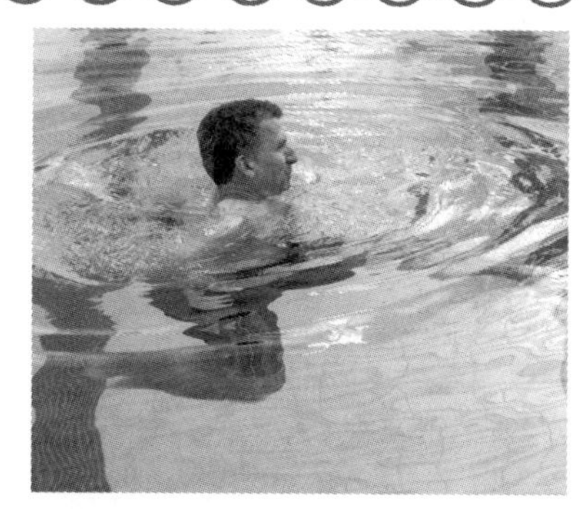

Start position.

FORM ISSUES

Pressing down with the arms. This issue occurs when participants attempt to pop higher out of the water by pushing their palms straight down during the power phase of the stroke. Their arms bend, followed by a push-down stroke close to their hips (as if attempting to do a press-up against the water). In my

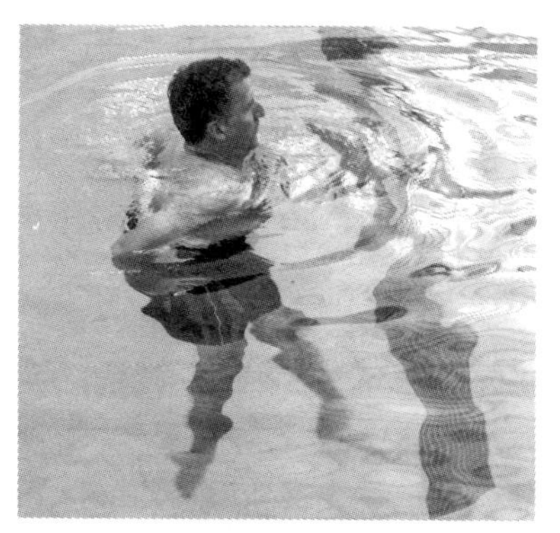

Power (pop) phase.

experience, this doesn't lead to any injuries, but you lose the full effect of the stroke. The core and upper body aren't as engaged as when using proper form.

Unbalanced power. This second issue is when participants are unbalanced—their legs drive too little and their arms drive too hard, thereby creating the pop-up with just their upper body. This is seen by the legs not reaching as far as they should, performing a shorter stroke. You can correct this issue by placing your hands on your hips and focusing on extending your legs far enough to generate the power for the pop-up only from the lower body.

PT POINTS

The Cross-Country Pop-Up still has the basic components of the Cross-Country, so please refer the corresponding PT Points on page 46.

HOW TO INSTRUCT FROM THE DECK

The key to this demonstration is to move at the same cadence that the participants would move in the water. Start slowly and deliberately at first, and then describe the increased power needed for the pop-up. By bending the planted leg and then extending it and raising up on your toes at the same time as the power phase of the opposite leg is being demonstrated, you can simulate the pop-up. Once the stroke is mastered, drills can be initiated without detailed demonstration.

Review of the shoulder concerns, especially with the backward reach and rotation of the arm, is strongly encouraged as this variation involves even more intense power. Useful terms and phrases include:

- Start off easy and get your range of motion first.
- Engage your core to ground your limbs.
- Equal power.
- Don't push harder with your upper body or lower body.

HOW TO USE THIS STROKE IN A WORKOUT

Use the Cross-Country Pop-Up in a main set or as the last set you do before transitioning from a warm-up to the main sets. It's a great stroke to use for longer sustained efforts as well as for short intervals.

BACKWARD CROSS-COUNTRY

While form remains mostly the same, this Cross-Country variation manipulates and changes the distribution of force within the power phase. The purpose of this stroke is to drive more power and intensity when the limbs are moving from the back position to the forward position in order to propel backward in the water, rather than keeping a balanced power as with a standard Cross-Country. Oddly enough, when performing this stroke, you may not even travel backward. Because the muscles that power the limbs from the back to the front are typically not as strong and well developed, travel backward may be minimal with this stroke. This is an aggressive and difficult stroke that requires increased power to drive the legs, working the quadriceps, hip flexors, abdominals, chest, and biceps. If you don't stabilize the spine at the very beginning of the power phase, the entire stroke will not achieve its full effectiveness. Again, think of the ungrounded open kinetic chain requiring additional stability through the core.

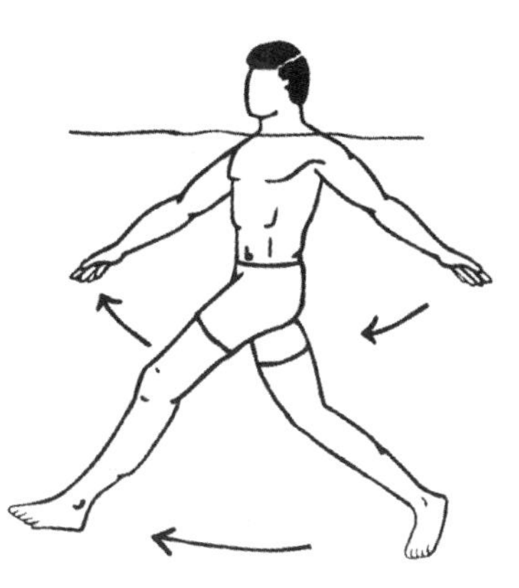

Stronger power from the back to the forward position.

This stroke integrates a complex and coordinated sequence that involves both the power and recovery phase within one stroke. This means your core needs to quickly shift from using the abdominals for the power phase to using the muscles primarily on the back side of the spine for the recovery phase.

This advanced stroke isn't recommended for beginners who may not be able to sufficiently engage the core. You also shouldn't do this if you have a compromised spine or lower back (see Cross-Country PT Points on page 46).

FORM ISSUES

There are several issues that can be seen with participants learning the Backward Cross-Country:

Unnecessary traveling. This is typically seen when you move backward through the water more quickly than necessary (aka, trying too hard to move). Your whole body may be tilting back in the water, which may cause you to augment the strokes by shortening your arm reach and pushing the water with your palms. The other common modification is to back pedal or scoop the water with your lower legs. To correct, maintain or return to an upright position, which will facilitate extension of the limbs farther behind, specifically eliminating the tendency to pedal/scoop. Also, remember that traveling backward isn't the primary goal.

Overreaching. You might try to gain more power from the stroke by overreaching with your legs, just like with the standard Cross-Country. This is typically seen through an overrotated pelvis/trunk to increase the backward reach of the legs, outside of the natural hip range and flexibility. As always, the stroke should follow your natural ROM. To recenter, place your hands on your hips to feel your hip/pelvis position, and avoid any rotating while performing the stroke with just your legs.

Lack of rotation. This is when a participant's torso doesn't rotate at all. With the vigorous Backward Cross-Country, it's crucial to have this slight rotation to facilitate core muscle contraction. To correct, a reminder and demonstration may be needed. *Note:* With a legs-only Backward Cross-Country, there's typically no torso rotation.

PT POINTS

When traveling in the less-common backward direction, the forces on the spine are significant in order to stabilize against the forces of the limbs. This intentional distribution of power requires exceptional strength, coordination, and stability of the core muscles, and structural integrity of the spine. If the spine isn't strongly stabilized when the limbs are driving in the forward direction, it will flex backward, possibly to the degree of hyperextension, most commonly experienced in the lower back. This also creates a stretching effect on the front of the body from the hips to the neck (backward bend), which is strenuous to overcome when transitioning to the recovery phase. The neck also tends to flex backward, triggering the natural response to pull the head forward, which can stress the neck muscles.

If you've had surgery at any level of the spine, injuries of the neck or lower back, or any abdominal surgery, take precautions. Please also review all the precautions stated in the Cross-Country (page 45), especially regarding the shoulder.

With respect to the lower limbs, the scooping or back pedaling motion of the legs (see Form Issues on page 67) puts excessive forces on the knee joint and can overwork the quadriceps muscles. As mentioned previously, the harder you push and the faster you try to move your limbs, the greater the resistance exerted by the water. The incorrect scooping or pedaling action in this powerful stroke is an open chain motion that isn't intended or recommended, especially if you've had knee surgery.

HOW TO INSTRUCT FROM THE DECK

Recalling the Cross-Country Pop-Up (page 65), as you demonstrate and verbally cue the intensity on the power phase of the stroke, it's important to keep one foot on the ground and simulate the movement by bending the planted leg and then extending and raising up on your toes. Useful terms and phrases include:

- Range of motion first, then power.
- Feel the quads as they drive forward.
- Feel your abs/core working.
- Slight rotation is okay.

HOW TO USE THIS STROKE IN A WORKOUT

I like introducing the Backward Cross-Country after performing extensive Water Run drills or the Breast Stroke Legs-Only that may have worked the hamstrings. I'd typically use it in a series of 30 seconds of an easier-effort Cross-Country, followed by 20 seconds of Backward Cross-Country, and repeat it three to four times.

BACKWARD CROSS-COUNTRY POP-UP

If the Cross-Country Pop-Up (page 65) and the Backward Cross-Country (page 66) weren't difficult enough, now try to combine them into one super-power effort: the Backward Cross-Country Pop-Up. This move simply increases the intensity to another level (or, as I like to think of it, "hell"). To perform this motion, initiate the Cross-Country, then transition into the Backward Cross-Country. To accomplish the pop-up, drive the limbs even more strongly toward the body while maintaining the form just as you did with the Cross-Country Pop-Up.

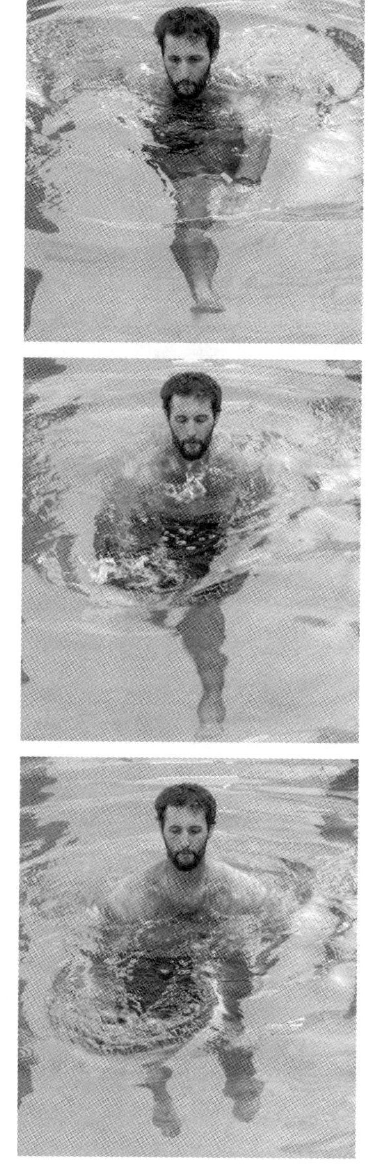

Start position leading into the backward power and then a pop-up.

FORM ISSUES

Overreaching. You may overreach to the rear and attempt a scoop to increase the power of the stroke. This is seen with increased knee bend at the start of the power phase to attempt to drive the scoop (similar to what may be seen in the form issues of the Backward Cross-Country on page 67). Your quadriceps will fatigue quickly. Although this isn't how the stroke should be performed, I haven't seen any injuries related to the stroke among healthy individuals.

PT POINTS

See PT Points for Backward Cross-Country on page 68.

HOW TO INSTRUCT FROM THE DECK

Start participants with the basic Cross-Country, reminding them to use equal power, then transition to the backward motion with the Backward Cross-Country before initiating the pop-up. Review the deck instruction notes for Cross-Country (page 47), Cross-Country Pop-Up (page 66), and Backward Cross-Country (page 68). Useful terms and phrases include:

- Range of motion first, then power.
- Feel the quads as they drive forward.

- You may not travel at all.
- Try to drive up and out of the water.

HOW TO USE THIS STROKE IN A WORKOUT

I recommend using this powerful stroke in a workout progression, starting with a Cross-Country, moving to a Backward Cross-Country, and then finishing with the Pop-Up over a 1 minute time frame. Repeat four or five times with recoveries.

CROSS-COUNTRY EX-BOX

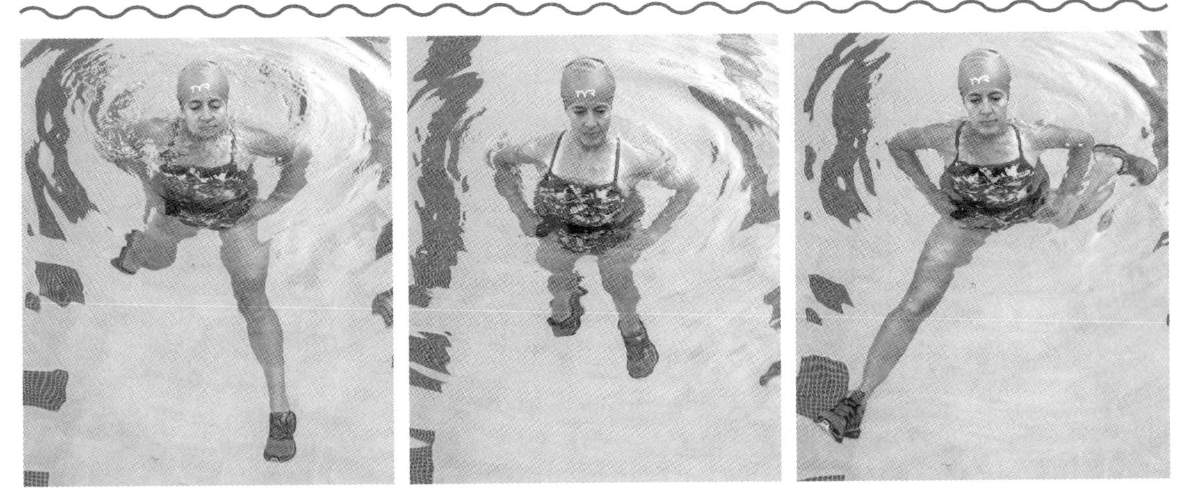

Start, follow-through with inward pull (power), and finish.

This advanced non-traveling stroke requires the mastering of the Cross-Country stroke (page 43). The Ex-Box adds an inward pull and outward push to the same Cross-Country leg motion for equal power phases. It's as if the legs were creating an "X" when the legs brush by each other just below the body. Then, as the legs drive away from the body, they finish about 10 to 12 inches to the right or left of the midline, which is a wider stance than the Cross-Country. This motion creates more work for the hip adductors and abductors.

This stroke is used to strengthen the legs, specifically the abductors and adductors. I prefer making the Ex-Box a legs-only stroke by keeping the hands on the hips or across the chest. It's possible to use the upper body, but some find the inward/outward motion awkward to coincide with the lower body, which could diminish the impact of the stroke. If that seems to be the case, switch to the legs-only variation.

FORM ISSUES

Overreaching. Overreaching or overextending the legs leads to power imbalances and form degradation because the legs reach farther than an individual's natural ROM. This is seen as the hip/pelvis of a single side overrotating (as in the case of an imbalance) or both hips/pelvis equally overrotating forward and backward. The stroke should follow a person's natural range of motion. If you place your hands on your hips and feel excessive hip motion, you're overreaching.

Bent knees. When your knees bend as your legs pass underneath, it decreases power and doesn't fully utilize the adductors and abductors. To correct, keep your legs extended throughout the stroke.

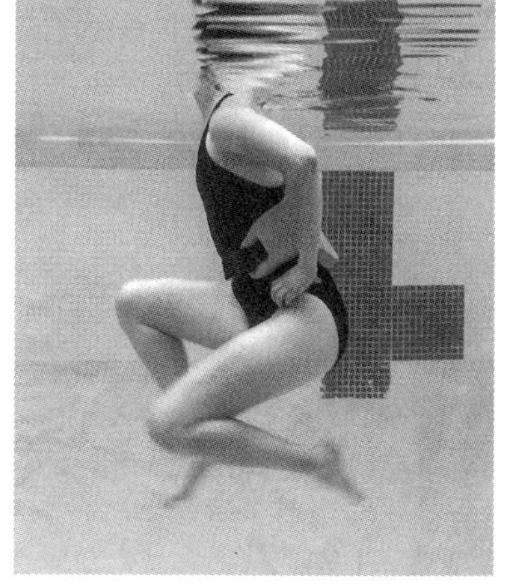

Do not bend your knees as your legs pass underneath.

PT POINTS

The motion of this stroke emphasizes the hip adductors located in the buttocks region and the adductors located along the inner thigh, which strongly push and pull the legs away from and toward the body. Soreness may be experienced when learning this stroke and developing these muscles.

HOW TO INSTRUCT FROM THE DECK

Begin with the basic Cross-Country before transitioning participants into the Ex-Box. Demonstrate in the same manner as the Cross-Country, with one leg planted while showing a front and side view of this new leg motion. You can also demonstrate the leg motion with the use of your upper body: Hold your arms out in front, facing the participants while showing the "X"— it's important to point out that you're using your arms to demonstrate the leg motion. The facilitator can also demonstrate/simulate the improper hip rotation if needed. Remind them that this stroke works the inner thighs (adductors) as well as the glutes (abductors). I usually receive a unanimous head nod when participants get it. Useful terms and phrases include:

- Keep the legs extended but not locked out.
- Smooth pull and push motion.
- Range of motion first, then power.

HOW TO USE THIS STROKE IN A WORKOUT

This is a stroke that shouldn't be introduced before mastering the Cross-County. I typically start a group in the Cross-Country and then have them perform power sets of the Ex-Box for 20 to 30 seconds at a time. I repeat the drill three to five times.

CROSS-COUNTRY WITH UPPERCUT PUNCH

Adding an Uppercut Punch to the Cross-Country creates an aggressive core workout. This variation of the Cross-Country is performed with more torso or trunk rotation to target and activate the abdominal obliques. The shoulder, chest, and biceps muscles are also highly utilized during the forward arm swings and additional elbow flexion. This is a non-traveling stroke but, with increased efforts, some backward movement may happen.

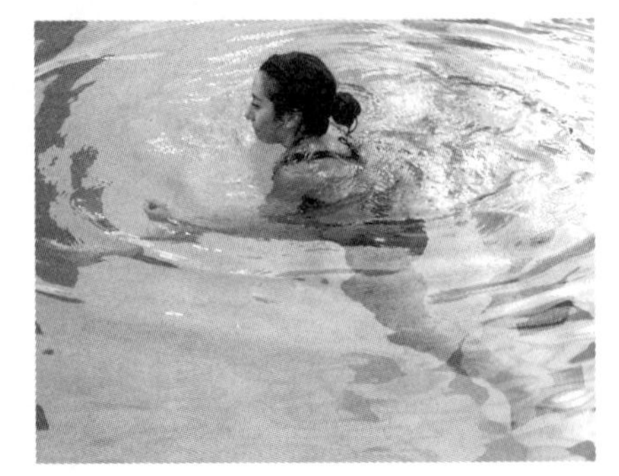

Cross-Country with Uppercut Punch.

Keep your arms in a palms-up, fisted position throughout the entire arm swing and punch as well as during the recovery. There's no shoulder rotation as in the regular Cross-Country when the arm moves from the front position to the back position because the palms don't rotate to face downward. The power phase begins with the arm behind the body and finishes as the hand crosses about 4 to 6 inches past the midline. Oblique activation occurs in this power phase. Although you use core muscles with the other strokes, the Cross-Country with Uppercut Punch may be the first time you experience the actual sensation of the abdominals engaging. The recovery phase occurs when the arm moves back to the start position.

There are two appropriate arm configurations: the straighter arm and the flexed arm. A straighter arm (which still maintains a slight bend in the elbow) makes the punch harder to execute due to the longer lever arm and increased water displacement. The more extended arm also slows the motion throughout the full arm stroke due to the increased resistance. The flexed arm uses more bend at the elbow and less rear reach with the hand, allowing the arm to move faster through the water due to decreased resistance.

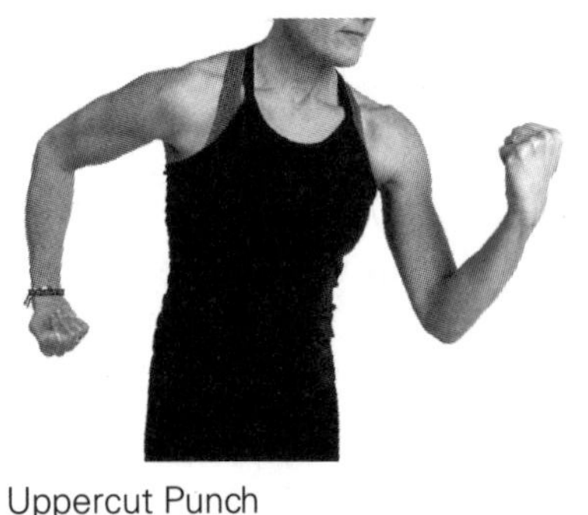

Uppercut Punch

Work your legs opposite to the upper body to accommodate the torso rotation, which specifically activates the abdominal oblique muscles. The torso rotation will create a slight midline crossover effect of the leg, both in front and behind you.

FORM ISSUES

Shoulder roll. When the upper body stiffens and doesn't rotate, it causes the elbow to lock out at the beginning of the punching motion. This looks nothing like a punch and is easy to spot as the shoulder rolls forward and appears to lead the punch motion (almost with a jerk), followed by the drag of the arm. This position exerts excessive pressure on the locked-out elbow as well as the shoulder joint and can deactivate the abdominals. In this situation, the shoulder muscles must compensate for lack of core activation, generating a highly ineffective punching motion. When you use the shoulder muscles as the sole driving force, you can experience shoulder pain. To correct, rotate your torso backward. This gives you the necessary reach and body position to effectively initiate the punch. When done correctly, expect to feel your obliques working.

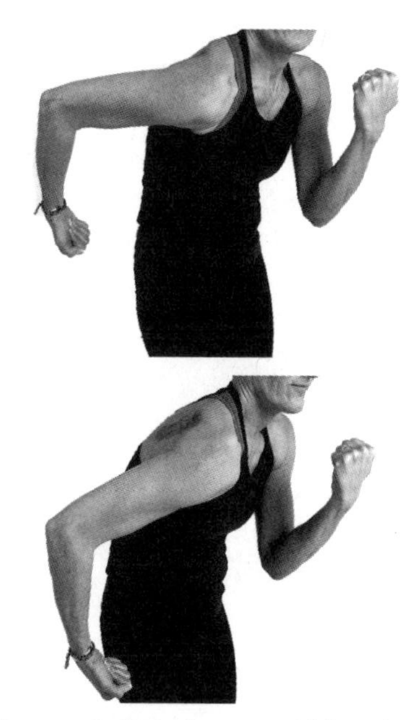

Incorrect start of uppercut (above) and excessive shoulder roll (below).

Lack of core engagement. When you try to gain more power with just the limbs (leaving out the abs), there may be a hesitation to rotate or have no rotation at all in the trunk. As mentioned, this stroke was intended for abdominal engagement to generate power and rotation. Remind participants to start the motion by first feeling their abdominal obliques before they initiate the upper cut punch; this should correct the issue.

Arm scoop. When the elbow is bent at more than a 90-degree angle, your arm is shortened and cuts through the water with too little resistance, which results in arm scooping. The biceps are only minimally activated, with minimal abdominal engagement. Simply extend your arm reach in the back position to feel the full benefit of this stroke.

PT POINTS

Review Cross-Country PT Points on page 46 and Punches PT Points on page 79, regarding shoulder concerns. If you've had shoulder surgery or shoulder dislocation problems, and/or biceps muscle or tendon issues, this backward reaching position and the action of punching forward against the water's resistance could be uncomfortable or may not be indicated.

If you do this stroke without core stability and proper alignment, the shoulder joint bears the brunt of the water's resistance. If you experience shoulder or upper arm discomfort or pain, check your form and reduce your intensity level if needed.

HOW TO INSTRUCT FROM THE DECK

Slowly demonstrate the trunk rotation and the punch with the arm, emphasizing the differences between a straighter or a bent-elbow position. Then demonstrate the trunk rotation and emphasize the abdominal engagement simultaneously with the leg motions. By breaking the stroke down in your demonstration, more participants will understand the various elements. When demonstrating the arm positions, reminding participants how to modify the power by changing the length of the arm. Start with the regular Cross-Country so participants can find their rhythm and range of motion before transitioning to the variation utilizing the Uppercut Punch. Useful terms and phrases include:

- Range of motion first, then power.
- Drive harder from the back to the front.
- Avoid driving through the shoulders.
- Feel your abs working.
- It's okay to rotate.

HOW TO USE THIS STROKE IN A WORKOUT

Because it takes several cycles of punching strokes to build power, I tend to use it for longer sets, those that are 30 seconds or longer. When performed correctly, this is a very tiring stroke.

KARATE KICK

In the Karate Kick, the limbs work opposite of one another, like the Cross-Country. However, the Karate Kick movements are higher in the water and are done with sharper execution. The legs drive forward and back reciprocally with a kicking motion rather than a sweep, with the foot held in a relaxed dorsiflexion (toes/foot up) throughout. In other words, as one leg swiftly kicks forward, the other leg simultaneously kicks backward with equal force and speed. This rapid motion requires significant core engagement to maintain postural integrity. Some forward travel may occur. The legs kick and then bend at the knees as the legs pass underneath, drawing up closer to the body; in some cases the knees will bend past 90 degrees.

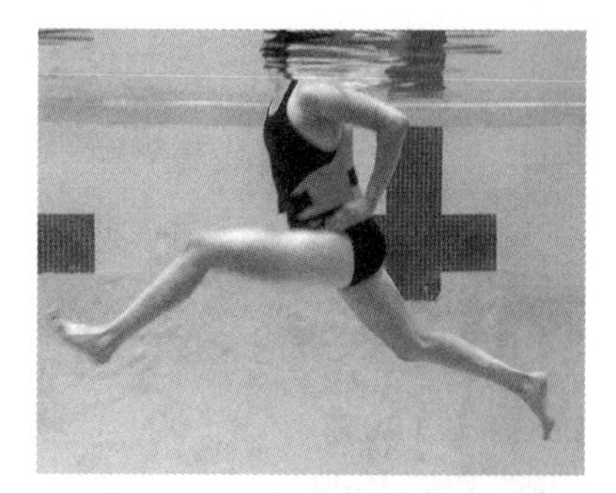

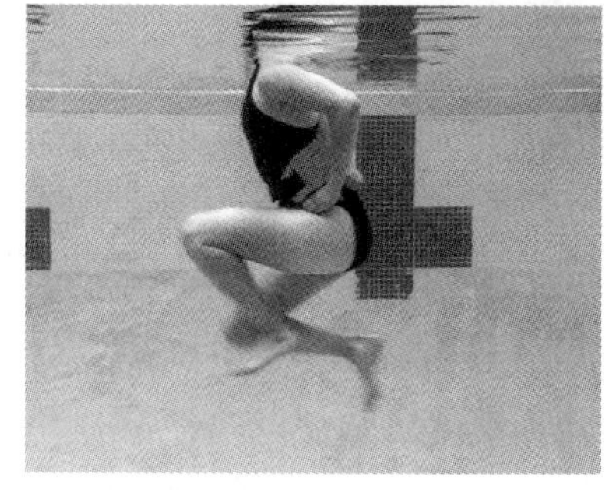

Legs extended and following through during the Karate Kick.

During the forward leg motion, the dorsiflexed foot engages the muscles of the core down to the quadriceps and the anterior tibialis (shins), and also stretches the hamstrings. During the backward leg motion, the hamstrings and gluteals are activated (imagine swiftly kicking shut a door directly behind you). If you lack hip flexibility, the backward motion is often challenging.

The upper limbs don't sweep as in the Cross-Country and don't drive as in the Water Run. Rather, the arm motion is intentionally left unspecified as it's based on the comfort of the participant.

Naturally, the arms will tend to move in the opposite-arm-to-leg motion, which helps power the drive of the lower limbs, or they're held on the hips to help isolate the movement.

This advanced move isn't recommended for anyone recovering from knee injuries or surgeries.

FORM ISSUES

Leg extension. Participants may keep the legs extended as they would with the Cross-Country throughout the entire stroke rather than kicking and bending the knees and drawing the legs up closer to the body. By providing a quick verbal reminder to pull the legs up toward the body when they pass underneath, the stroke should become more accurate.

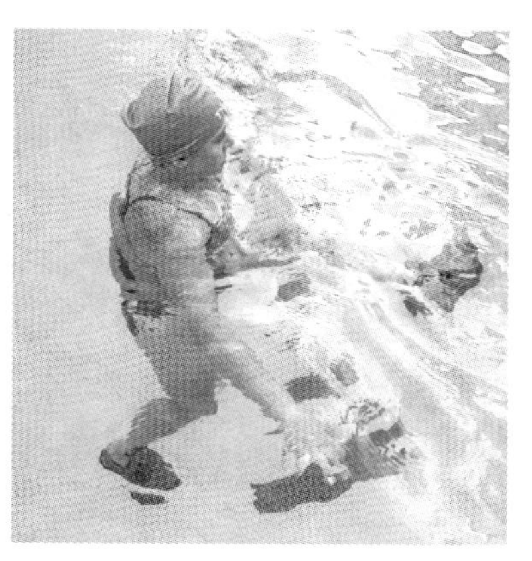

Incorrect: legs drop down rather than tuck under and are not extending back.

Downward kick. A common issue is when the kick is directed downward, below the individual, instead of driving back behind the torso. To perform uniform kicks forward and backward, start with less leg extension and drive a bit lower in the water, focusing on equivalent leg motions. Gradually bring the legs higher as you slowly increase the cadence while maintaining proper form.

PT POINTS

The Karate Kick's rapid leg extension in both directions can be strenuous on the knee. If you've had knee surgery, including but not limited to treatment of ACL/PCL, meniscus, or any type of reconstruction, or you suffer from instability of the knee joint, it's highly recommended that you consult your physical therapist or physician before attempting this move.

If you begin experiencing pain in the knee or hip joints, decrease intensity and the extension of the legs to a more comfortable level.

HOW TO INSTRUCT FROM THE DECK

I've found that most participants will attempt the Karate Kick by using the Cross-Country motion rather than a punctuated kick. Therefore, the demonstration needs to involve the motion of one leg kicking forward, with the foot dorsiflexed, followed by the leg bending then sliding directly under the body and driving back, while cuing that this isn't the Cross-Country motion. You can even demonstrate each of the two strokes and how they differ so participants can see the distinction. Use a quicker cadence demonstration so participants can see that the stroke

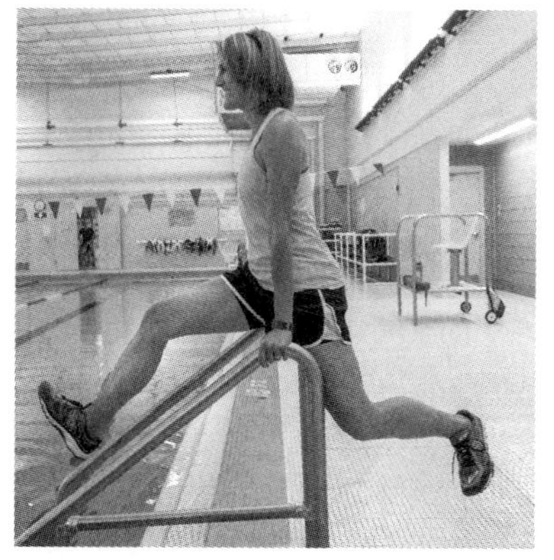

Karate Kick using the handrails on the pool ladder.

is performed more rapidly. Utilizing the handrails on the pool ladder can help with this demonstration. I'll even suggest that they pretend they're performing this stroke in three to four feet of water, as to imagine not kicking the floor of the pool. Useful terms and phrases include:

- Range of motion before power.
- Focus on the kick back.
- Drive the foot forward. Feel the shins working.

HOW TO USE THIS STROKE IN A WORKOUT

This stroke is intended for a shorter interval, from 15 seconds up to 30 seconds. I have participants start off slowly and then increase their effort in order to maintain the proper form and ROM.

PUNCHING: THREE VARIATIONS

The first time punching in a pool was written about was in the 1960s as a publicity stunt by the late (and great) Muhammad Ali, complete with photographs taken by Flip Shulke. The published image is of Ali standing submerged underwater in a fighting stance. Although the photos were a stunt, exercises using a punching action in a pool are realistic as well as challenging and intense.

A deep-water punch is relatively straightforward and uncomplicated. However, because of the significant core involvement requiring focus, inexperienced participants may find it difficult to perform. This is why punching is introduced in this advanced section.

The three punches in this section—the Straight-Shot, the Uppercut, and the Hook—require torso rotation and increased core strength/coordination to ground the punch and to synchronize contractions with the rapid alternating arm motions. The punch should be delivered rapidly and intensely, so shorter intervals of 15 to 30 seconds at a time are optimal. The hands are always in a fisted position.

The punch works numerous muscle groups from the abdominals, chest, lats, deltoids, biceps, and forearms. The key to planting a punch is to engage the core strongly to stabilize and use trunk rotation to assist in driving the arm forward with force and power. The recovery occurs when the arm returns to the back position. Even in this recovery phase, the arm must move backward very quickly against the water's resistance, adding to the core stability requirements as well as providing additional conditioning and strengthening effects.

If the drive of the arm comes from the shoulder (rolling the shoulder forward) and the abdominal component is neglected, this creates jerking-type motion, as discussed in the Cross-Country Uppercut Punch Form Issues on page 79). The power-generating component is the work of the abs to help drive the arm forward, as if propelling the punch through an object, such as when connecting with a punching bag. When working with a heavy bag, you're not trying to slap—or stop short—at the bag; rather, you drive your force through the bag. With water, although there isn't an object to connect with, the action is the same.

The lower limb motion for the punches is all the same, therefore it will be explained at one time here. Start with a Water Run, and then find your own rhythm or pattern that works to complement the punch being performed. Regardless of the leg movement pattern, it should be synchronized with the upper body. With the Hook, you may find that the legs naturally spread a bit wider in the water to mimic the wider arm movement. In addition, adjusting the forward lean from the upright body position can increase core engagement.

For clarity purposes, we'll introduce the three punch strokes, then explain the Form Issues, PT Points, and How to Instruct and use them in a workout.

STRAIGHT-SHOT PUNCH

Start the Straight-Shot Punch with the hand held just to the side of the body several inches below the armpit/chest, thumb pointing toward the body. Engage the core and drive one arm straight out in front, finishing the stroke with an almost fully extended arm about 4 to 8 inches below the water's surface. Since you're driving quickly with this stroke, the water should churn significantly. I refer to this as making "white water."

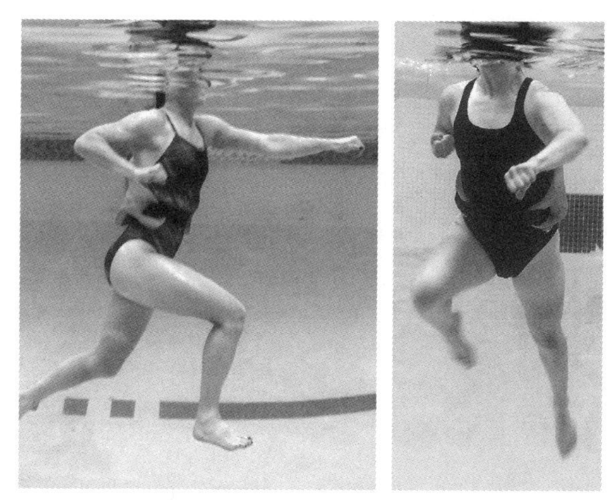

Straight-Shot Punch

UPPERCUT PUNCH

Start with the hand held slightly behind the hip, palm up and fisted with additional torso rotation. The torso rotation allows the arm to reach back more at the start of the punch and still maintain a bend at the elbow. The Uppercut drives forward while the elbow flexes, as with a biceps curl, and finishes at about the midline under the surface of the water. The recovery phase occurs when the arm returns to the start position. This punch can be used with a more or less flexed elbow. The longer the arm (i.e., lever), the more drag occurs when the arm is driving from the back position to the forward position. If you choose to extend the elbow, the hand at the start position will be slightly lower than hip level. The increase in drag will require more core involvement and more effort. Important: Refer to Form Issues in the Cross-Country Uppercut Punch (page 72).

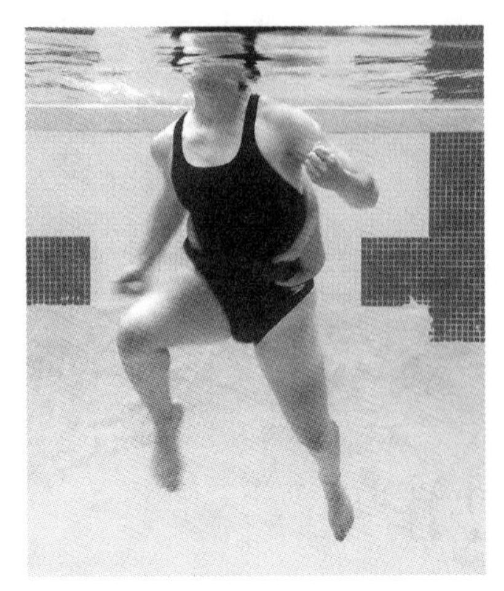

Uppercut Punch

HOOK PUNCH

The Hook looks similar to the Uppercut; however, there's additional torso rotation and the arm is extended more and slightly behind the participant, palm up and held in a fist, approximately 12 to 14 inches away from the body. The Hook drives forward while the elbow flexes (as with a biceps curl) yet maintains its position away from the body. The power phase finishes at about midline, several inches under the surface of the water. The recovery phase is when the arm returns to the start position. The abdominal muscles, especially the obliques, are engaged in the power phase to increase core stability.

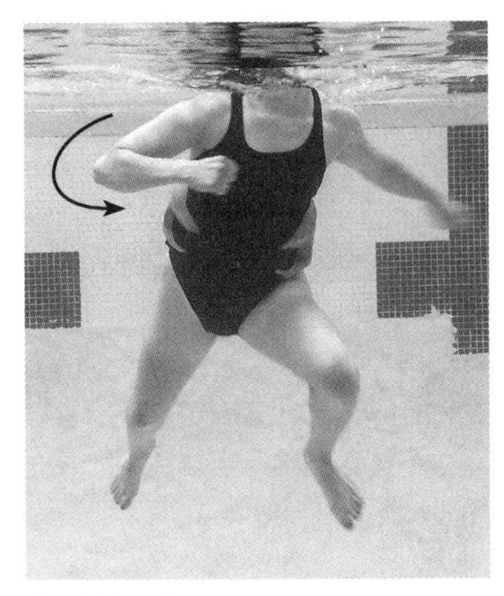

Hook Punch

Since the arm is farther away from the body during the Hook's power phase, there's additional drag. The longer the arm's reach, the more strenuous effort is required to complete the forward motion. The degree of elbow flexion depends on which muscles you want to target. For additional chest and biceps work, drive the arm forward with a more flexed elbow.

FORM ISSUES FOR ALL PUNCHES

Lack of power. If you're punching like you're swatting at gnats—arms flailing forward or driving from the shoulder—it means nothing's happening. There's no power, no drive. Lack of power is also caused when you don't initiate the punch in the correct start position. Remember to rotate your torso and start in the correct place to maximize the power.

PT POINTS FOR ALL PUNCHES

The vigorous, rapid movements of the arms with all of these punch variations requires conditioning of not only the core and shoulder muscles but also the biceps, which bends the elbow and also brings the arm upward and forward. You may find that these muscle groups need additional strengthening before they're able to provide the stability and power to sustain this stroke at a fast pace. Pain and the inability to maintain proper form and/or technique are signs that you're unable to tolerate this level of intensity. Check your form and reduce your effort level as needed.

The Hook will be the most challenging of these variations due to the wider arm swing away from the body with a more extended elbow.

If you try the Uppercut Punch without sufficient core stability and proper alignment, the shoulder may roll forward and has the potential to expose the shoulder joint to the brunt of the water's resistance. The shoulder joint isn't designed to function with this added force when dragging your arm through the water. See Form Issue Shoulder Roll in Cross-Country with Uppercut Punch (page 72) for the description of this problem and the technique for correction.

If you've had shoulder surgery or shoulder dislocation problems, and/or biceps muscle or tendon issues, these punching motions and the rapid, intense action against the water's resistance could be uncomfortable or may not be indicated. Consult with your therapist or physician.

HOW TO INSTRUCT FROM THE DECK

Demonstrate all three punching strokes slowly so participants can see where to start and finish each stroke, including the length of the reach. Verbally emphasize the power phase. Typically, I introduce one punch, have the group perform it, then lead into the next (and so forth). This allows the group to gain mastery of each stroke.

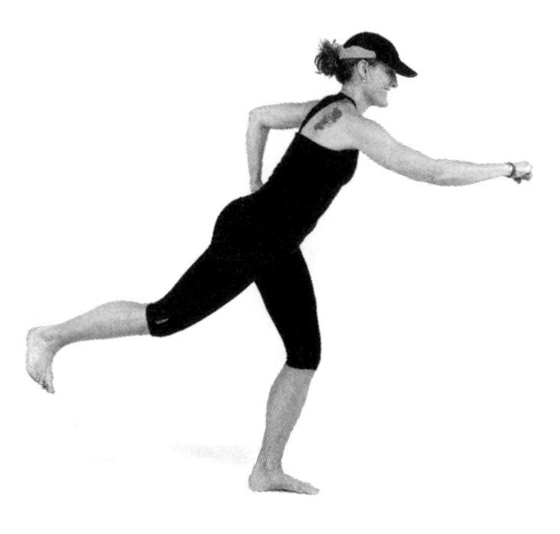

Demonstrating the Straight-Shot Punch.

The Punch is intended to be intense and delivered with a rapid cadence; it's not meant to be performed slowly. That said, the extended arm won't be able to punch through the water at the same speed as the arm with a more flexed elbow. Take time to demonstrate a straighter or more bent arm to show that angle of the arm affects the resistance and would change the difficulty and effort needed for the stroke. Useful terms and phrases include:

- Avoid driving through the shoulders.
- Feel your abs working.
- Make white water (for the Straight-Shot Punch).
- It's okay to rotate for more power.

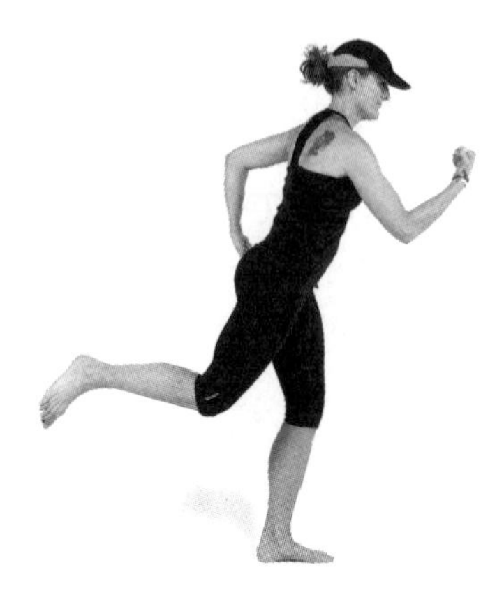
Demonstrating the Uppercut Punch.

HOW TO USE THIS STROKE IN A WORKOUT

I recommend using the punch strokes in series of speed work. Ideally, I'd perform one stroke for 15 to 20 seconds, followed by an equal recovery. Then continue the same timed sets for the next two strokes. To really feel the impact of this drill, I'd then repeat it three to four times!

ARMS-ONLY PUNCH

Removing the use of the legs during any of the three punch strokes requires the core to engage even more in order to provide the stability for the power of the punch. This unifies the muscle function of the core and the upper body. Once you try this, you'll soon discover it's not as simple as it may sound.

Start with any of the punches using your full body to gain power and momentum. Transition gradually into eliminating the leg movement; relax them and let them hang or cross the ankles. This slow transition will allow the participant to increase the core/oblique engagement in order to be able to deliver the punch with proper form at the same intensity. This core-centric focus of the Arms-Only Punch creates fatigue even faster, so plan on shorter-duration sets when first introducing this stroke variation.

FORM ISSUES

Lack of power. If you relax your core/abdominals, you lose the punch's power. Reintroduce the leg work to help engage the core, then try it with just the upper-body movement once core engagement is re-established. Transition participants back and forth between a full-body punch and Arms-Only to help them maintain the intensity of this powerful stroke.

Breakdown of form. When participants stop using their legs, the actual punch form may fall apart. If the stability provided by the core muscles is insufficient due to either fatigue or the inability to engage them properly, participants won't be able to maintain the punch form. This will be seen as the arms starting to flail. Have them reintroduce their legs and re-establish the core; this allows for the transition back to the proper stroke form and the can begin again.

HOW TO INSTRUCT FROM THE DECK

Demonstrate the punch strokes as you previously learned and verbally cue the participants to gradually relax their legs while keeping their core engaged. Remind them that there's much more abdominal engagement, and because of this it's okay to transition back to using their legs at any time for a "break." Useful terms and phrases include:

- Feel your abs working.
- Make white water (for the Straight-Shot Punch).

HOW TO USE THIS STROKE IN A WORKOUT

As with the previous recommendation, the Arms-Only Punch is designed for short durations. I suggest using this stroke in a progression drill, performing each stroke for 20 seconds—each starting with a Water Run, moving to a Full-Body Punch, then on to Arms-Only. Repeat this 1 minute set three to four times after a 30-second recovery between each.

CHAPTER 6

The HIT Workout

> *"When planning an aquatic workout, follow the same principles as those of land-based exercises. Frequency, intensity, and volume must be considered...you should structure the workouts with specific goals and organization."*[44]

When talking to individuals about training or working out in a pool, the immediate reaction is boredom—I've literally seen the light go out of their eyes. Merely the mention of spending an hour to an hour and a half in a pool drains the enthusiasm out of athletes. This doesn't have to happen.

There are many stroke variations that can be used to develop workout sets in order to use the pool to cross-train.[45] Just like other types of training activities, pool workouts can have distinct goals: a day to work endurance and another for speed. Therefore, similar principles apply. As suggested by the *Aquatic Fitness Professional Manual,* knowing what you want from your workout is key before you dive into the pool.[46] If the workout is a rest day, keep the effort at recovery level. If you want to work on speed, focus on intervals in the pool.

"Deep water running performed as continuous and interval training promotes an improvement in agility and dynamic balance, in the strength of upper and lower limbs, in the flexibility of lower limbs, and of cardiovascular fitness."[47]

It's important to change it up in any workout, whether in the water or on land. For example, runners shouldn't do speed work every day—this produces muscle soreness, fatigue, breakdown, and overtraining. Experienced cyclists, swimmers, cross-country skiers, and other sprint and high-endurance athletes plan a variety of effort levels within a weekly training regimen. So when deep water exercises are used to supplement or replace a daily land workout, match it with the effort level to its corresponding land activity.

This chapter covers a universal approach to HIT training, starting with understanding how to find your correct water-based heart rate. Details on workout design and training variations follow, ending with a few sample HIT workouts. Remember to be mindful and intentional about the use of deep water training. It can be as difficult as interval work performed on land.

FINDING YOUR HIT TARGET HEART RATE FOR WATER EXERCISE

Your target heart rate is the aerobic range you should work in for your best workout results. This is typically 55 to 85% of your maximum heart rate. If you exercise above the target heart rate, you're straining too much; if you go under, you're not getting the most out of your workout. Athletes and sports enthusiasts use their target heart rate to get the optimal benefits from their workouts. But athletes doing water exercises for the first time always assume that their heart rate would behave the same in water as it does on land. They're then quite surprised to find out that their effort in water feels different and their heart rates are significantly lower (see How Water Affects Heart Rate on page 24). This next section will show you how to determine the correct hydro heart rate using two methods: 1) an aquatic deduction method, and 2) a cadence drill method with a modified rate of perceived exertion (RPE) Borg scale.[48]

AQUATIC DEDUCTION METHOD

While the Karvonen Heart Rate Scale is used to find land-based heart rate, I use the Kruel equation for finding water-based heart rates.[49] The Kruel calculation adds an additional calibration to account for the hydrodynamic properties of a submerged body in water.[50] In order to find this aquatic deduction, take a 1 minute resting heart rate on land and submerged.[51] Once you have the figures, subtract the water heart rate from the land heart rate, and that's your deduction.

To attain the most accurate deduction figure, do this test on two other mornings at about the same time each day, then use the average of the three. Using myself as an example, my mid-morning 1 minute resting heart rate is 82 on land (in a heated pool room) and 64 in the pool. Therefore, my aquatic deduction calculation would be: 82 – 64 = 18. My aquatic deduction is 18.

Next, you'll need your morning resting heart rate (your heart rate when you first wake up; taken three days in a row to find your average) as well as your age. My morning resting heart rate is 49 and I'm 50 years old.

With this data, the below calculations show both the use of Kruel's water-based equation and Karvonen's land-based equation.

Equation for Kruel Aquatic Heart Rate with Deduction:

$$220 - \text{Age} - \text{Resting Heart Rate} = X$$

Using my figures:

$$220 - 50 - 49 = 121$$

$$\frac{(121 - 18) \times (85\%) + 49}{= 136 \text{ Target Aquatic Heart Rate}}$$

$$(X - \text{Aquatic Deduction}) \times (\%\ \text{intensity}) + \text{Resting Heart Rate} = \text{Target Aquatic Heart Rate}$$

Equation for Karvonen Method (land-based heart rate):

$$220 - \text{Age} = \text{Age Predicted Max Heart Rate}$$

$$= \text{Target Heart Rate}$$

Using my figures:

$$220 - 50 = 170 \text{ Age Predicted Max Heart Rate}$$

$$\frac{(170 - 49) \times (85\%\ \text{intensity}) + 49}{= 152 \text{ Target Heart Rate on Land}}$$

$$(\text{A.P. Max Heart Rate} - \text{Resting Heart Rate}) \times (\%\ \text{intensity}) + \text{Resting Heart Rate}$$

Using Karvonen's method, my target heart rate effort of 85% is 152. But when using the aquatic deduction scale developed by Kruel, my target heart rate effort at 85% intensity is 136, a significant difference of 11.2%. I'd need to know this difference when performing any type of intensities in the water, and so will your participants. Think about this: If my heart rate was 152 in water, it would equate to 169 on land (adding back that 11.2%). That's much higher than what I should be doing; it's outside of my safe target heart rate zone. Now coaches can work and challenge their athletes outside of this safer heart rate zone. However, I suggest that most fitness enthusiasts remain in the 55 to 85% target heart rate zone. Unless you're able to test each participant using the full Kruel deduction method and scale, a safe suggestion to a group of new participants would be to err on the conservative side and simply deduct 20 to 30% from the land heart rate for an equivalent water heart rate.

If you're tracking your heart rate, the table on the next page will demonstrate why it's important to know the difference between heart rates when on land and when immersed in water so you don't overexert yourself in the water. The table below demonstrates this variability in heart rate using my personal statistics and deduction percentage of 11.2%.

LAND HEART RATE	WATER HEART RATE
120	107
130	115
140	124
150	133
160	142
170	151
180	160

CADENCE DRILL METHOD & RATE OF PERCEIVED EXERTION (RPE) SCALE

Another way of establishing a target heart rate uses a cadence drill. This method is relatively easy to conduct and can help participants judge exertion levels. The chart below correlates a land-based running cadence (minutes per mile) with a cadence rate (how many single leg rotations completed per minute) in the water. The corresponding rates produce essentially equivalent exertion levels based on a five-point rate of perceived exertion (RPE) scale. For example, the exertion level of a 10-minute-mile pace on land would correlate to a water-run cadence of 85, considered to be a RPE of 4, or hard.[52] Consider using a metronome to help maintain specific cadence rate.[53]

Water and Land Rate of Perceived Exertion[54]

RPE	WATER RUN (Leg circle per minute)	LAND RUN (Minute per mile)
1	Very light (< 50)	Slow walk (< 21)
2	Light (50–60)	Medium-paced walk (15–20)
3	Somewhat hard (60–75)	Fast walk/jog (< 15)
4	Hard (75–85)	Hard Run (5–10)
5	Very hard (> 85)	Very hard run (> 5)

In order to try out the RPE or cadence rate methods, you'll need to first re-calibrate a standard heart-rate work-zone chart (this chart matches intensity levels to a corresponding heart rate range) with your heart rates reduced by the conservative deduction of 20 to 30% to take into consideration the effects of deep water. I find that the best way to measure heart rate in water is to perform an activity then stop and immediately perform a six-second count of your pulse. Waiting any longer, you won't achieve a correct reading: your heart rate drops down very quickly due to the effects of water and you will get a falsely low exercise rate. Compare the six-second water heart rate to your adjusted work-zone chart to give you an estimate of the workout intensity. By taking your heart rate in this manner several times and paying attention to how your body feels, you'll understand the relation of your heart rate to the level of exertion. This will give you an estimate of the workout intensity. This will also allow you to establish a correct RPE scale for water training. Standard RPE scales such as the Borg method use a numbering system of 1 to 10 or 6 to 20, with the numbers representing the perceived effort.[55] Lower numbers represent little to no effort; upper numbers represent very hard or extremely hard efforts.

When working with novices, it's important to discuss the RPE scale as well as explain the interval training concept, including effort percentages. This will help them learn how to judge their effort levels during any given workout. Most deep water interval-training workouts are performed at a moderate to intense levels. It takes practice to become familiar with your body's responses so that you can gauge your efforts accurately. This ability will gradually increase with time.

With a lowered heart rate in water, the perception of one's true exertion level can be deceiving and you may not sense exactly how demanding a workout is. Because of this, novices can work too hard before they're ready to do so. This results in muscle fatigue, soreness, and potential injury. Monitor your efforts! The various signs that you're working too hard are very similar to those on land: your face is red, you're unable to catch your breath, you have difficulty breathing, and/or you feel nauseated. By using RPE, heart rate percentages, and cadence rate, you can cue intensities by adjusting to your participants' needs.

When I work with a group fitness-type class, I vary my cues to include RPE, effort percentages, and descriptors such as, "This next set will require a very strong effort. You'll be breathing very hard and you'll feel that it's difficult to keep the effort. This should be 85% of your overall max effort." Another favorite is, "If you feel cold, you're not moving enough." Or, "If you can breathe through just your nose, you're not working at 85% effort." The last cue is also a good tool to help people find their target heart rate in the pool. Typically, the need to breathe through the mouth is a good indication of working at 80% or above (whether in the water or on land). Today, with new heart rate monitors geared for water training, it's easier to monitor heart rates when deep water training.

DESIGNING YOUR OWN HIT WORKOUT

As a coach and trainer, I've developed a thought process about how a workout will affect an athlete, especially if they have injuries that need to be addressed. I consider what they need to gain from that workout (such as targeted strengthening of weak muscle groups, or protection of a specific body part) and what the specific goal is for that day (for example, recovery vs. interval). If you're an individual adopting HIT in your training regime, the key is to develop a workout that effectively targets your personal fitness goals. If you're an instructor designing a workout for a group, the workout design may be more universal.

Developing a deep water workout can seem complex. My intent is to simplify this process and provide tools to help you develop your own system. The workout structure can fall into one of the following areas:

- Balanced workouts for full-body training
- Targeted workouts for upper or lower body
- Workouts for sports-specific training

BALANCED WORKOUTS FOR FULL-BODY TRAINING

A balanced workout is my typical "go-to" set for a group training session that involves a variety of athletes and fitness levels. The goal of a balanced workout is to train the entire body, not focus on one aspect of the body or another. I find most athletes enjoy the challenge of this type of workout as they'll be shown a new way to move their bodies, build on their current fitness base, or enhance their overall training for their land-based sport. The work performed in a balanced workout may not always be sport-specific (e.g., runners may not just be doing the Run), but it does introduce athletes to stroke variations that could expose weaknesses that they didn't know existed.

TARGETED WORKOUTS FOR UPPER OR LOWER BODY

An upper- or lower-body-focused workout can be ideal to strengthen specific muscle groups or to correct an imbalance. For individuals recovering from an injury, any part of the body can be protected from overwork while still using the unaffected limbs. After I injured my shoulder in a bike accident, I used the pool to continue training. Although I couldn't work my upper body with the same intensity as my lower body, I could still continue with interval training, core exercise, and recovery work without compromising the rehabilitation efforts on my upper body. Likewise, the same can be done for the lower body, such as with a sprained ankle.

It's important to remember that workouts that focus on the upper or lower body require considerable core stabilization; the more an area is isolated, the more the core is necessary to stabilize the body. As fatigue may set in faster, frequent recoveries may be needed during any of the sets performed.

WORKOUTS FOR SPORT-SPECIFIC TRAINING

Sport-specific training deserves a book of its own. For any sport, think how individuals train and move within that sport. Now consider which strokes might simulate or complement these movements and how particular muscles can be targeted.

People typically think of deep water training only for runners, so triathletes and runners are the ones most often drawn to the pool. However, as I've mentioned with examples of high-level athletes from figure skating and hockey to baseball, water is a platform for all.

TRAINING VARIATIONS

> *"Increased speed of motion increases the energy expenditure of movement only if you keep exactly the same range of motion. If you decrease the range of motion when you increase tempo, energy expenditure is reduced."*[56]

Training variations, or changes in tempo or speed, help make your workouts interesting and keep you challenged and engaged. The great thing about training in the water is that it's immensely versatile; as you've seen in the progression from basic to advanced strokes, even a slight change in effort or muscle engagement or a shift in movement can quickly change the focus or intensity of any stroke.

This section will review how to utilize and plan a warm-up and cool-down effectively with different strokes, and contain discussions on the benefits of traveling or stationary work. All of these will include exercise intensity levels, including concepts such as the steady-state and progressive efforts. This section will also review additional types of training drills such as the Break-Out Stroke or the use of Eddy Drill. The actual workout sets are in the last section of the chapter.

WARMING UP, RECOVERY, COOLING DOWN, & STRETCHING

Each of these components are important aspects of a workout. However, if you take a quick look at the sample workouts, the warm-ups, cool-downs, and stretches aren't included for each workout. They were intentionally left out—not because they're unimportant but because they're typically conducted in the same manner regardless of the nature of main workout. I've elected to explain them separately in order to provide more detail.

To reiterate, warming up, recovery/cooling down, and stretching are highly beneficial, so please don't eliminate them from your regimen. Refer back to this section to ensure you incorporate them effectively.

WARM-UP

The sole purpose of a warm-up is to prepare the body for the upcoming activity. It's a critical component that, if not done, can affect the entire interval session that follows. If the muscles and cardiovascular system aren't prepared for the intensity that follows, they won't perform maximally to achieve the desired results. There's also a higher chance for muscle breakdown, fatigue, and injury. The warm-up is a great time to incorporate the strokes that are planned in the main workout set. This will allow the participants the opportunity to learn the stroke, experiment with the new motions, and develop muscle memory (the ability to perform motions without necessarily thinking about them, similar to riding a bike).

Most exercises in deep water training can be used for warm-up, cool-down, or intervals. However, a few strokes are better suited for easier efforts. I prefer strokes that allow the body a larger ROM rather than ones with tighter movements. The Breast Stroke, Cross-Country, Water Run (at an easier effort or with an extended reach), and the Water Walk all are great strokes for warming up. A warm-up will typically last 5 to 10 minutes, with the last few minutes spent working in progressive efforts to transition into the upcoming higher-intensity interval sets. The progressive and repetitive sets are usually 45 to 60 seconds in length with short recovery between each.

By starting with strokes that use large motions and gradually working in quicker moving strokes, participants tend to perform with cleaner form and smoother transition when moving into increased power. Conversely, by starting with a fast Water Run or a Karate Kick, for example, participants may tighten up and then maintain this same rigid form throughout the remainder of the class.

RECOVERY/COOL-DOWN

Recovery is an integral part of an athlete's training, whether in the water or on land. Recoveries come in various ways within a training regimen, from those that occur within an interval set to those that happen at the end of a workout (called cool-down) and those that fall within a training program each week. The cool-down will be the third type of recovery described.

> *"...the recovery period is most often a form of active rest, as opposed to true rest in which all activity is ceased."*[57]

The first type of recovery is the phase during the actual motion being performed. The recovery phase follows a stroke's power phase and is composed of the movement to return the limb to the starting position. For example, in the Water Walk, the power phase is when you drive the arm from the forward to back position, while the recovery phase is when you move the arm forward back to the catch.

Another type of recovery occurs within a repetition or set—a brief rest period (while still performing a stroke) built into each set that allows the body to recover and be ready for the next drill—it's the nature of interval training. This is an active recovery that's meant to be short and timed just like the interval; too long of a recovery between sets lessens the impact of the interval and the purpose behind training in this method.

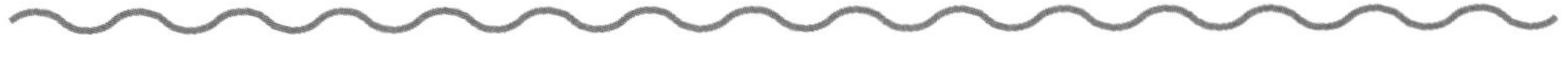

DEEP WATER TRAINING AS RECOVERY

Deep water training doesn't have to always be at high, interval efforts; it can be used purely for a recovery workout within a weekly routine. When I first introduce hydro exercises as a recovery method to my athlete clients, they're a bit skeptical, especially since their only experience with deep water had been an intense training session. A couple of my cycling athletes were very surprised by how relaxed and stretched out they felt after recovery training in the pool. If you're on a recovery day, perform one of the suggested workout sets starting on page 97 but use lower intensity levels and longer recovery durations. The reduced intensity will allow you to stretch a bit more when performing certain strokes, such as the Cross-Country.

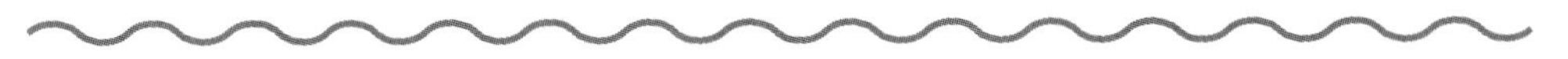

The third type of recovery, also called a cool-down, occurs once the main workout session is completed. This is very similar to the purpose of performing a warm-up, but in reverse. You're working at lower intensities and moving from more of an aerobic effort to a very easy effort, allowing your body the time to return to its pre-workout state. This recovery may be a bit shorter than land-based recoveries because water temperature, characteristics of the athletes/participants performing the exercises, as well as the types of exercises and intensities performed can all affect the speed that the body will resume its pre-workout state.

The temperatures of many athletes with low levels of body fat will drop more quickly than the average person. Typically, the higher the percentage of body fat, the warmer the participant. Therefore, pool temperatures below 80 degrees will have some participants shivering rather quickly, making it important to keep athletes moving so that they continue to generate some body heat, even during recovery. If you choose to combine stretching with the recovery component of the workout, a light Water Run or Water Walk between stretches performed on the wall is ideal. If this active recovery can't happen, participants may be more comfortable only cooling their temperature down in the water and then stretching on land once dry.

Last, the fourth type of recovery occurs within a long-term training program. Training repetitive high intensities can cause muscle breakdown and injury; therefore, recovery workouts should be incorporated into training each week/month. By doing so, the body (muscles/cardiovascular system) has the chance to recover and be prepared to work hard again. I'd say that the number-one issue I see with new participant to any sport is their lack of understanding of the importance of recovery. They assume that if they can't perform with intensity each day, it's due to lack of ability or fitness, so they try to train even harder. The results are muscle fatigue, soreness, injury, overtraining syndrome, or illness, all of which then removes them from the sport they've fallen in love with—for weeks or months at a time.

STRETCHING

The best ways to stretch after a deep water exercise cool down is to utilize the pool wall. Using the wall will allow participants to hold on with their hands to achieve a more relaxed mode of stretching while taking advantage of the buoyancy effect. Stretches are held for 30 to 60 seconds, similar to land-based stretches. Keep in mind that a majority of the movements in the strokes also incorporate stretching, so the requirement for stretching isn't the same as after most land-based trainings. Plan to focus the final stretches on the parts of the body that weren't already stretched during the workouts. Below are descriptions of four types of stretches I like to perform after a full-body workout.

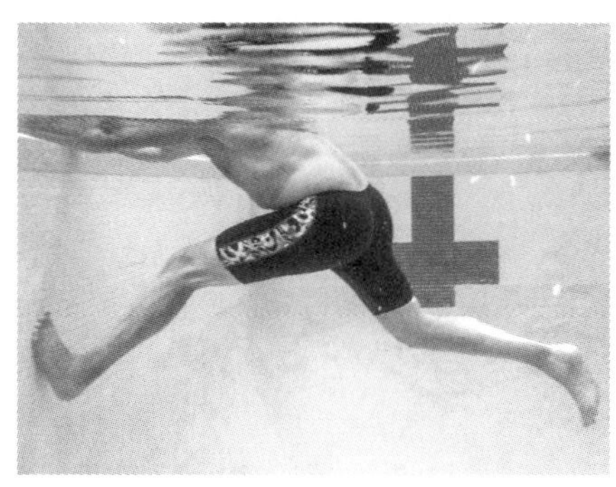

Full-Body Stretch

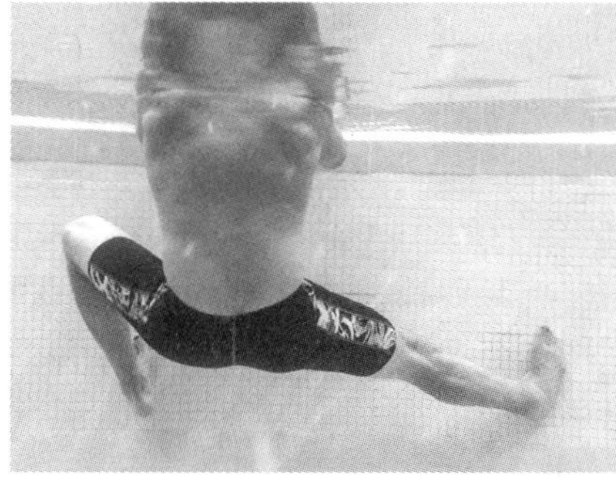

Runner's Stretch

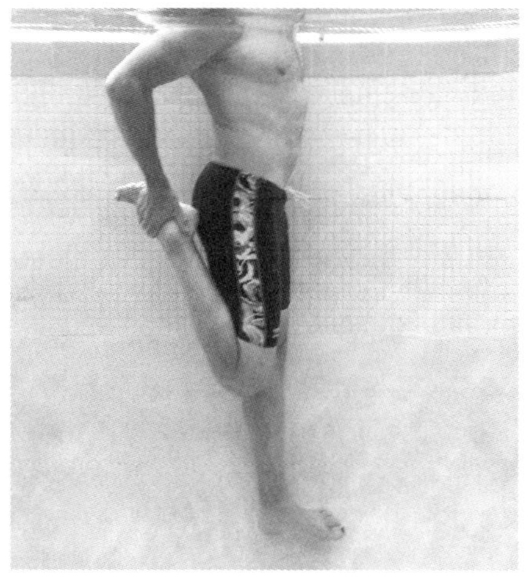

Quadriceps Stretch

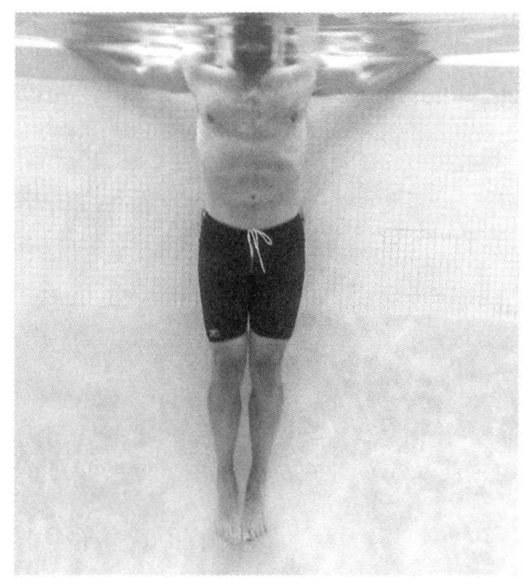

Figure-Head Stretch

The Full-Body Stretch is similar to downward dog in yoga except performed in the pool. One leg is on the wall of the pool (foot flat on the wall with the knee locked or with a slight bend) while the other leg is lifted and stretched behind the participant. This move stretches the triceps, latissimus dorsi, hip flexors, hamstrings, and calves.

The Runner's Stretch is performed with the legs "standing" on the pool wall, bending one knee at a time in order to focus stretching the opposing adductor.

The Quadriceps Stretch also uses the wall to brace and targets the quadriceps and hip flexors.

The Figure-Head stretches chest and biceps muscles. It's very relaxing and is typically saved for the last stretch. Then stretch your arms out at your sides and allow your shoulders to roll out while resting the outward side of your hand on the wall of the pool. If you grip the pool wall, you only stretch the deltoids, not the intended chest and biceps. The key is to relax your body and let it hang along the wall of the pool; your feet may even rest on the pool wall. Due to the position of the shoulder joint, consult with your health provider or therapist before trying this stretch if you've had any type of should injury and/or surgery.

DEVELOPING THE MAIN SET

The Main Set, designed primarily for interval training, is the crux of this training platform. Most coaches are familiar with this type of training, as are group fitness instructors who teach indoor cycling, HIIT, Tabata workouts, or any other interval-based workout with times sets. If you don't have a background in this type of training, an explanation of the purpose/rationale, benefits, and the structure of intervals will follow.

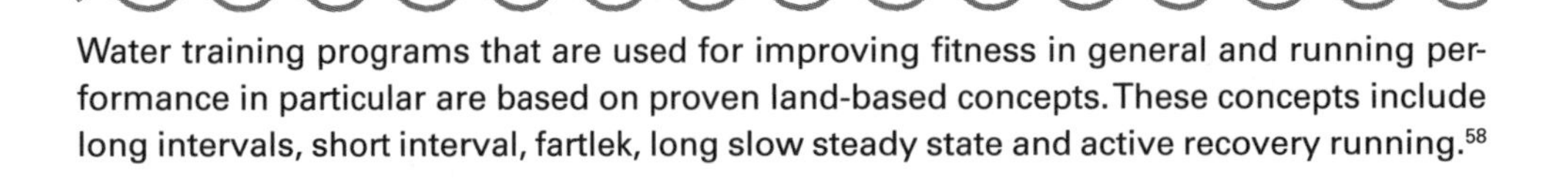

Water training programs that are used for improving fitness in general and running performance in particular are based on proven land-based concepts. These concepts include long intervals, short interval, fartlek, long slow steady state and active recovery running.[58]

Interval training (long, short, and fartlek) is a type of training that involves changing intensities between a harder and an easier effort, with the ultimate purpose to improve overall endurance. The goal of interval training is to see improvements over weeks/months, primarily the ability to work longer and harder while maintaining a lower heart rate. Interval work also produces a higher caloric burn than an aerobic effort. This means higher caloric consumption is needed for athletes and the opportunity for increased weight loss (if desired).

Typically the hard efforts are anaerobic, and the easier efforts are at a recovery or working level (aerobic). All intervals don't need to be at an intense effort; it depends on the participant and the desired outcome for the workout on that given day day.[59] In many cases, interval durations follow set ratios. For example, 1:1 means the same length of interval as recovery, 1:2 means recovery time is twice that of the interval, 1:3 means recovery is three times that of the interval time. Intervals can be long (e.g., up to 5 or 10 minutes) or short (e.g., 15 seconds). As previously mentioned, the length of the intervals and recoveries are all based on the work that needs to be done in the training session.

It's important to note that intervals typically shouldn't be conducted every day but rather on non-consecutive days, as rest between intense workouts is important in promoting optimum performance. For some individuals, more than one day of recovery between intense interval workouts may be necessary. Typically, the older you are and the earlier you are in your fitness-building process, the more recovery days you may need; it truly depends on the individual, their general health and fitness level, and their response to interval training. If you find that your energy (the effort you need to perform a harder effort) just isn't there when you try to perform interval work every other day, you may need to include another day of lighter-effort (recovery) work.

TRAVELING VS. STATIONARY

As you've learned, a majority of the strokes are performed in a stationary position, but a few can be used with some travel involved. I've found that fast travel encourages participants to think that moving more quickly through the water equates to a harder effort with more intensity. But, in many cases, moving quickly means that the participant isn't working as hard, and instead is manipulating the stroke (making it easier) in order to travel more quickly.

If a person is traveling, it's important to understand whether they're performing the stroke correctly or not. For example, you may look down in the water during the Water Run and see a participant reaching out in front farther and wider than others, almost performing an underwater swimming type of stroke. If you see this, understand that although they're moving faster, it's with less effort and intensity. When participants are traveling, even slightly, while performing a stroke that's intended to be stationary, remind them that they're not balancing the force of their limb movements in the forward and backward directions and that they may be working at a lower intensity.

STEADY STATE VS. PROGRESSIVE STATE

A steady state means you remain at a constant speed/effort while a progressive state means you gradually increase speed/effort over the duration of the set. Both can be used with any effort desired, depending on where they fall within the workout set or your training regime. The purpose of a steady state is to teach pacing at specific efforts.

I typically use the steady state anywhere between a strong (75%) to moderately uncomfortable (85%) effort. I find that an 80 to 85% effort for several minutes, especially with inexperienced athletes, is the hardest to maintain both physically and mentally. When I watch experienced athletes performing a steady-state effort, I can see them almost mentally "lock" into it as the effort is bringing them to a familiar race pace. It will take many sessions before I witness this in any individual not accustomed to any type of racing or hard sustained efforts.

The biggest problem when introducing a steady state is that individuals new to the pool or to training have difficulty maintaining higher steady efforts for any given time. When working with a large group of non-athletes, a 5- to 10-minute set becomes excruciating, physically and psychologically. Therefore, longer sustained sets should be reserved for an experienced group of athletes. How do you know if the set was too long for your group? You'll actually witness a slow decline in effort, with the form falling apart as well. By simply starting newer trainees with shorter 1- to 2-minute sets and then slowly building the duration to longer sets over several weeks, you can train a group to sustain longer steady-state efforts (if desired). If you're working with a mixed group of participants (perhaps ranging from seasoned athletes to those less familiar with intense training), then work the two slightly differently. For example, by having the less-experienced individuals recover for 15 to 30 seconds after each sustained minute and having the experienced group continue the steady-state effort for 5 minutes, you can easily have a variety of fitness abilities in one group.

For a progressive effort, the drill will usually start with an easier aerobic effort and then increase to the target effort. These building efforts teach participants how to hold back and maintain an effort, and then how to push harder when they're ready. By mastering their own energy expenditure, participants will be able to effectively manage their efforts through a short set or an entire workout (or a race). New participants may push harder than they really should, resulting in not being able to recover sufficiently to start the next repetition. This drill will teach them how to discover their abilities as well as their limits, then they can to work confidently and effectively within any given set.

Using a progressive build doesn't mean that every set should push to an all-out effort at the end; it depends on the desired outcome. For those individuals who tend to fall apart as they push harder, I find pacing drills, such as the steady state, as well as progressive drills helpful in addressing this issue.

BREAKOUT STROKES

A breakout on land is when an athlete is working at a steady state during an event or training and then, at any point, exerts more effort to pass another athlete. To pass a competitor (or target), a runner must use more effort, but not so much that she exhausts herself as she'll need to return and maintain her steady state. A breakout stroke (BOS) is typically for a given period of time, usually 5 to 20 seconds. The purpose of a breakout stroke is to teach the maintenance of proper form while transitioning between various efforts. Inexperienced participants often work too hard during interval transitions and can't resume a steady state. Instead, they shift into a lowered effort state or a full recovery mode due to fatigue. An analogy for this would be if you'd passed your target while running but couldn't keep up your original pace while in front, which can result in you being passed by your target shortly afterward. The best suggestion is to ask participants to only work slightly harder during the breakout stroke than during the steady state.

The breakout stroke can be of varied lengths and performed with varying strokes. It also doesn't have to be the same stroke for the duration of the set. As an example, a group performing a Water Run for 5 minutes at a low threshold effort could perform 10 to 20 seconds of a High Knee as the breakout stroke. Before introducing the breakout stroke, I usually prepare participants with progressive drill sets. By doing so, participants will feel the various efforts throughout the progression and can determine the right intensity for the breakout stroke.

The ability to balance pushing oneself without overexerting is a learned skill. This is something most speed/endurance coaches work into training sessions, so it transfers smoothly into deep water intervals.

EDDY DRILL

The Eddy Drill works with and against the water resistance and turbulence created by the participant's motions to challenge and train for power and acceleration. In HIT, an eddy is the movement of water, or current, that occurs behind a participant's moving body, like a mini whirlpool, and doesn't affect the athlete unless they turn and move directly into it (i.e., turbulence). In a pool workout, all participants are creating eddies behind them when they're traveling. This swirling current can literally pull the participants together, or it can be used to challenge your athletes, which is what I choose to do with the Eddy Drill.

The higher energy demands of turning and running into (or pushing "against") the wall of swirling water (i.e., the eddy forming behind the participant) is the crux of this drill. Introduce the eddy by having all participants face the same direction while performing a Water Run, making sure they're spread out enough not to catch up to each other. Once you start the clock, you'll call out "turn" about every 5 seconds (meaning a 180-degree U-turn) and have them continue with the Run. The key to making this drill extremely challenging is timing—turning the participants just at the moment that the water starts to give way (i.e., the pressure of the water begins to ease up and starts moving with them, rather than against them). After waiting for 7-plus seconds, you'll lose the intended effect of trying to "run upstream." The participants should technically be performing the eddy in the same six-foot space because of the repeated 180-degree turns, but the desire to move beyond that given space is very strong and most participants will lean forward in their run to almost a dog paddle. Therefore, be sure to keep their form intact with constant reminders.

When creating sets that include the eddy, recall that they're strenuous. A 30-second drill is hard; performing it for an entire minute is extremely fatiguing. However, for an even more challenging variation, you can use group dynamics to create even more water turbulence. I enjoy having my participants attempt to tag others by pairing them up—one facing the back of the other—about five to six feet apart. It's extremely hard to catch the other person, but being chased by another will make them work harder, not to mention the added water turbulence created by other participants.

SAMPLE WORKOUTS

Now it's time to put all the pieces together and give a few of these workouts a try, whether you're an individual exploring HIT or a trainer, coach, or fitness instructor. You have knowledge of the merits of deep water exercise and the foundation of all the strokes, as well as an appreciation for heart rate responses and exertion/effort levels. You've been provided guidance for interval-based workout design and training variations, including the equally important warm-up, cool-down, stretching, and recovery. Additional enhancements to a workout have been included, such as Breakout Strokes and the Eddy Drill.

Following are 10 balanced workouts that are designed for a general group of participants. Each workout can fit into a one-hour training, with the main set (interval portion of the workout) approximately 40 minutes in length and the remainder of the time spent in warm-up, cool-down, and stretch.

Workout 1: Full-Body Focus

Between each drill perform a recovery or working effort.
Run for 1 minute.

	EXERCISE	DURATION	SETS (TIME)
	Warm-Up		
DRILL 1 Total time: 6:00	Progressive to 85% effort: Cross-Country *(page 43)* Water Walk *(page 55)* Water Run *(page 38)*	1:00 on/off	1 each (6:00)
DRILL 2 Total time: 4:30	Eddy Drill *(page 95)*: Water Run *(page 38)* at 85% effort	:30 on/off :45 on/off 1:00 on/off	1 each (4:30)
DRILL 3 (repeat 3 times) Total time: 10:30	Rotate between each: Punch—any *(page 76)* High Knee *(page 48)*	 :20 on/off :15 on/off	 3 (2:00) 3 (1:30)
DRILL 4 Total time: 3:00	Water Walk *(page 55)* at a steady state 80% effort	1:00 on/:30 off	2 (3:00)
DRILL 5 Total time: 4:30	Repeat Drill 2		
DRILL 6 Total time: 3:00 Total time: 4:30	Repeat Drill 4		
DRILL 7 Total time: 4:00	Cross-Country with Uppercut Punch *(page 72)*	:30 on/off	4 (4:00)
DRILL 8 Total time: 10:30	Repeat Drill 4		
	Cool down and stretch on the wall		

Workout 2: Five Pyramids

In each pyramid, perform the numbered exercises in a 1, 2, 3, 2, 1 pattern. Rest 1+ minutes between each pyramid.

	EXERCISE	DURATION	SETS (TIME)
	Warm-Up		
PYRAMID 1 Total time: 6:40	1. Water Run with Closed Hand *(page 38)*	:15 on/off	3 (1:30)
	2. High Knee *(page 48)*	:20 on/off	2 (1:20)
	3. Breast Stroke *(page 59)*	:30 on/off	1 (1:00)
PYRAMID 2 Total time: 7:10	1. Cross-Country *(page 43)*	:45 on/off	1 (1:30)
	2. Punch—any type *(page 76)*	:20 on/off	2 (1:20)
	3. Flutter Kick *(page 51)*	:15 on/off	3 (1:30)
PYRAMID 3 Total time: 7:50	1. Karate Kick *(page 74)*	:15 on/off	3 (1:30)
	2. Cross-Country with Uppercut *(page 72)*	:25 on/off	2 (1:40)
	3. Water Walk *(page 55)*	:45 on/off	1 (1:30)
PYRAMID 4 Total time: 7:10	1. Backward Cross-Country *(page 66)*	:45 on/off	1 (1:30)
	2. Hook Punch *(page 78)*	:20 on/off	2 (1:20)
	3. Straight-Shot Punch *(page 77)*	:15 on/off	3 (1:30)
PYRAMID 5 Total time: 8:30	1. Water Run *(page 38)*	:15 on/off	3 (1:30)
	2. Cross-Country Pop-Up *(page 65)*	:30 on/off	2 (2:00)
	3. Breast Stroke *(page 59)*	:45 on/off	1 (1:30)
	Cool down and stretch on the wall		

Workout 3: 10-Drill Total Body with Breakout Strokes (BOS) Between each drill perform a recovery or working effort. Breast Stroke for 1 minute.			
	EXERCISE	**DURATION**	**SETS (TIME)**
	Warm-Up		
DRILL 1	Cross-Country *(page 43)* with BOS Cross-Country Pop-Up *(page 65)*	:30 on/off	4 (4:00)
DRILL 2	Water Run *(page 38)* with BOS Hook Punch *(page 78)*	:15 on/off	5 (2:15)
DRILL 3	Cross-Country *(page 43)* with BOS Flutter Kick *(page 51)*	:20 on/:30 off	4 (3:20)
DRILL 4	Water Run *(page 38)* with BOS High Knee *(page 48)*	:20 on/:30 off	4 (3:20)
DRILL 5	Cross-Country *(page 43)* with BOS Water Run *(page 38)*	:15 on/off	5 (2:30)
DRILL 6	Water Run *(page 38)* with BOS Karate Kick *(page 74)*	:30 on/off	3 (3:00)
DRILL 7	Cross-Country *(page 43)* with BOS Cross-Country with Uppercut Punch *(page 72)*	:30 on/off	4 (4:00)
DRILL 8	Water Run *(page 38)* with BOS Straight-Shot Punch *(page 77)*	:15 on/off	5 (2:30)
DRILL 9	Cross-Country *(page 43)* with BOS Backward Cross-Country Pop-Up *(page 69)*	:30 on/off	4 (4:00)
DRILL 10	Eddy Drill *(page 95)*: Water Run *(page 38)*	1:00 on/off :45 on/off :30 on/off	1 (2:00) 1 (1:30) 1 (1:00)
	Cool down and stretch on the wall		

Workout 4: The Repeater

Between each drill perform a recovery or working effort.
Water Walk for 1 minute. Suggest a reverse hand.

	EXERCISE	DURATION	SETS (TIME)
	Warm-Up		
DRILL 1 (repeat 3 times) Total time: 18 minutes	Rotate between: Progressive Water Run *(page 38)* Cross-Country Pop-Up *(page 65)*	:45 on/:15 off :15 on/off	4 (4:00) 4 (2:00)
DRILL 2 (repeat 4 times) Total time: 8 minutes	Rotate through three strokes: Water Run *(page 38)* Karate Kick *(page 74)* Breast Stroke—legs only *(page 62)*	:20 on/off	1 (2:00)
DRILL 3 (repeat 3 times) Total time: 12 minutes	Rotate between: Flutter Kick *(page 51)* High Knee *(page 48)*	:20 on/off :15 on/off	3 (2:00) 4 (2:00)
DRILL 5 (repeat 2 times) Total time: 8 minutes	Rotate between: Uppercut Punch *(page 78)* Eddy Drill *(page 95)*: Water Run *(page 38)*	:30 on/off :30 on/off	2 (2:00) 2 (2:00)
	Cool down and stretch on the wall		

Workout 5: Progressive Pyramid

To perform the pyramid, the entire set is 1, 2, 3, 4, 3, 2, 1. Each exercise is progressive in nature. After each numbered set, recover with a Water Walk for 1 to 2 minutes.

	EXERCISE	DURATION	SETS (TIME)
	Warm-Up		
DRILL 1	Cross-Country *(page 43)* Water Run *(page 38)* Breast Stroke *(page 59)* Cross-Country Pop-Up *(page 65)* Water Run—legs only *(page 38)*	1:00/:45 off	1 (8:45)
DRILL 2	Breast Stroke *(page 59)* Water Run—with fists *(page 38)* Cross-Country with Uppercut Punch *(page 72)* Water Run—slice hands *(page 38)* Cross-Country Pop-Up—legs only *(page 65)*	:40 on/:30 off	1 (5:50)
DRILL 3	Karate Kick *(page 74)* Cross-Country Ex-Box *(page 70)* High Knee *(page 48)* Backward Cross-Country—legs only *(page 66)* Water Run *(page 38)*	:25 on/:15 off	1 (3:20)
DRILL 4	Hook Punch *(page 78)* Flutter Kick *(page 51)* Uppercut Punch *(page 78)* Flutter Kick *(page 51)* Straight-Shot Punch *(page 77)*	:15 on/:10 off	1 (2:05)
	Cool down and stretch on the wall		

Workout 6: Mixed Bag of Tricks

After each numbered drill, recover with a Water Walk stroke for 1 minute.

	EXERCISE	DURATION	SETS (TIME)
	Warm-Up		
DRILL 1	Breast Stroke *(page 59)* with a BOS Backward Cross-Country *(page 66)*	:30 on/off	4 (4:00)
DRILL 2	Water Walk at 80% effort *(page 55)*	1:00 on/off	1 (2:00)
DRILL 3	Water Run with BOS Sprint Run *(page 38)*	:15 on/:25 off	6 (4:00)
DRILL 4	Cross-Country *(page 43)* with BOS Cross-Country Pop-Up *(page 65)*	:20 on/:20 off	6 (4:00)
DRILL 5	Reverse Hand Breast Stroke: at 80% *(page 59)*	1:00 on/off	1 (2:00)
DRILL 6	Eddy Drill *(page 95)*: Water Run at 85% effort *(page 38)*	1:00 on/off :45 on/off :30 on/off	1 each (4:30)
DRILL 7	Water Run *(page 38)* with BOS Karate Kick *(page 74)*	:20 on/:20 off	6 (4:00)
DRILL 8	Repeat Drill 2		
DRILL 9 (repeat 4 times) Total time: 8:00	Perform each stroke within one set: Water Run *(page 38)* Punch *(page 76)* High Knee *(page 48)* Flutter Kick, change hand and leg variations for more complexity *(page 51)*	:15 on/off	1 (2:00)
DRILL 10	Cross-Country *(page 43)* with BOS High Knee *(page 48)*	:20 on/:20 off	6 (4:00)
DRILL 11	Repeat Drill 5		
	Cool down and stretch on the wall		

Workout 7: Quick Turnover

After each numbered drill, recover for 30 seconds to 1 minute before starting the next drill.

	EXERCISE	DURATION	SETS (TIME)
	Warm-Up		
DRILL 1	Eddy Drill *(page 95)*: Water Run *(page 38)*	:30 on/:30+ off	4 (4:00+)
DRILL 2 (repeat 3 times)	High Knee *(page 48)* (recover :30 to :45 between each set)	:20 on/off	3 (2:00)
DRILL 3 (repeat 3 times)	Rotate between Punch *(page 76)* and Water Run recovery *(page 38)*	:20 on/:20 off	2 (2:00)
DRILL 4	Progressive Repeats: Water Run *(page 38)* Cross-Country *(page 43)* Breast Stroke—fisted hands only *(page 59)*	1:00 on/:30-:45 off	2 (9:00+)
DRILL 5	Repeat Drills 3, 4, and 1		
	Cool down and stretch on the wall		

Workout 8: Repeating Pyramids

In each pyramid, perform the numbered exercises in a 1, 2, 3, 4 (3, 2, 1) pattern.
Recovery Breast Stroke for 1 to 2 minutes between each pyramid.

	EXERCISE	DURATION	SETS (TIME)
	Warm-Up		
PYRAMID 1 Total time: 14 minutes	1. Cross-Country *(page 43)*	1:00 on/off	1 (2:00)
	2. Karate Kick *(page 74)*	:45 on/off	2 (3:00)
	3. Punch—various types *(page 76)*	:30 on/off	3 (1:00)
	4. High Knee *(page 48)*	:15 on/off	4 (2:00)
PYRAMID 2 Total time: 14 minutes	1. Water Run *(page 38)*	1:00 on/off	1 (2:00)
	2. Cross-Country Pop-Up *(page 65)*	:45 on/off	2 (3:00)
	3. High Knee *(page 48)*	:30 on/off	3 (1:00)
	4. Punch—various types *(page 76)*	:15 on/off	4 (2:00)
	Repeat Pyramid 1 or 2		
	Cool down and stretch on the wall		

Workout 9: Long and Short

After each numbered drill, recover for 30 seconds.

	EXERCISE	DURATION	SETS (TIME)
	Warm-Up		
DRILL 1	Punch—various types *(page 76)*: As the duration becomes longer, intensity drops	:20 on/off	1 each (4:40)
		:30 on/off	
		:40 on/off	
		:50 on/off	
DRILL 2	Breast Stroke *(page 59)* Cross-Country *(page 43)* Water Walk *(page 55)*	1:00 on/off	1 (6:00)
DRILL 3	Repeat Drill 1: Change stroke to Karate Kick *(page 74)*		1 each (4:40)
DRILL 4	Repeat Drill 2		1 (6:00)
DRILL 5	Repeat Drill 1: Change stroke to Run *(page 38)*		1 each (4:40)
DRILL 6	Repeat Drill 2		1 (6:00)
DRILL 7	Repeat Drill 1: Change stroke to Cross-Country *(page 43)*		1 each (4:40)
DRILL 8	Repeat Drill 2		1 (6:00)
DRILL 9: PYRAMID Total time: 6:30	1. High Knee *(page 48)*	:15 on/off	3 (1:30)
	2. Flutter Kick *(page 51)*	:20 on/off	2 (1:20)
	3. Punch—various types *(page 76)*	:25 on/off	1 (:50)
	Cool down and stretch on the wall		

Workout 10: Rapid Fire After each pyramid drill, recover for 30 seconds to 1 minute with any stroke (time not figured in overall posted time).			
	EXERCISE	**DURATION**	**SETS (TIME)**
	Warm-Up		
DRILL 1	Water Run with BOS Water Run *(page 38)*	:30 on/:30 off	4 (4:00)
DRILL 2: PYRAMID (repeat 5 times) Total time: 31:30	1. High Knee *(page 48)*	:15 on/off	3 (1:30)
	2. Punch—various types *(page 76)*	:20 on/off	2 (1:20)
	3. Karate Kick *(page 74)*	:25 on/off	1 (:50)
DRILL 3	Water Run with BOS Water Run *(page 38)*	:20 on/:30 off	4 (3:20)
	Cool down and stretch on the wall		

APPENDIX

Teaching HIT & Getting Others Hooked

Looking back, I am amazed at how much we learned without even noticing it.

—Azar Nafisi, *Reading Lolita in Tehran*[60]

The process of learning to teach, wherever the classroom may be, is not a quick one. It needs to be nurtured and cultivated and is never-ending. I love the quote by Julia Child, "*You'll never know everything about anything, especially something you love*," as I can't help but reflect that every time I work with someone in the water or on land, *I learn.* I learn new ways to cue and terms to use when correcting improper movements (and more creative approaches to address the issues). Most of all, I learn more about myself as an educator, coach, trainer, and athlete.

I've been developing and evolving my teaching methods for years. Therefore, I could write chapters on the matter. I feel that my background as a credentialed teacher has always helped me in the fitness world. The understanding of class management and how to generate lesson plans naturally supported me in developing effective, progressive training programs. However, telling you everything I know about how to teach isn't the intention of this book. There are many certification programs and education systems that can help you become a coach, trainer, or fitness instructor. My recommendation is if you need training in this area, seek certification through an accredited source (e.g., ACE, NASM, ACSM, AEA, or USA Triathlon, to name a few). The intention of this chapter is to put the first six chapters to use, whether you're a credentialed or certified instructor or not.

This chapter won't just guide you through hydro interval training (HIT) instruction—it will also provide simple teaching tips for group exercise dynamics in the pool, managing a variety of fitness and skill levels during a single class, and participant/instructor interaction, as well as give you guidance as to what types of additional tools you can use.

INTRODUCING PARTICIPANTS TO HIT

Teaching participants in a completely suspended environment is very different from shallow water classes. More verbal cues and imagery are required to assist participants to effectively perform the appropriate movement pattern.[61]

Teaching, in any venue, is a skill that one must take time to learn and improve upon. I've seen and experienced some ineffective coaches who thought they could coach simply because they once were athletes. This is a fallacy. Being a good instructor is something that's honed over time with practice and training, trial and error, and a passion for educating and teaching. All these concepts apply to instructing or coaching in the deep water as well.

Training in the deep water is weird. Yes, I said "weird." When performing this type of training for the first time, I've seen participants' emotions range from laughter to frustration to anger due essentially to a change in coordination experienced as lack of control of their body's motion in the water. For most of them, this is a completely new activity. New movements, new environment—it could be considered a whole new "sport."

The first few training sessions are vital to keeping a participant motivated and interested. This initial adjustment phase can take three to five sessions, with some participants able to reach the intensities desired during this period, while others take more time. Once the ability to execute the stroke without any major form issues is achieved and the understanding of water dynamics is integrated, participants can begin to apply increased efforts. Encourage patience by reminding them to follow a simple principle: "Form before power."

As a coach, being aware of the form imbalances and why they're happening will help you work with your athletes. Consider educating your group about the changes they'll feel with their center of gravity, the lack of body (kinesthetic) awareness brought on by the unfamiliar environment, and their need to literally "relearn" normal body movements.

It's important to remind participants regularly that it will take time to master this new environment. Don't assume that they'll adapt without your frequent input. Even if you're working with athletes who typically feel attuned to their bodies, this guidance and information can lessen the frustration and aggravation and keep them engaged during the learning process. Remember, there are no mirrors so they can't "see" what they're doing.

The role of a coach is to consistently train the group for mastery of the strokes and then build in the challenge of increased intensities and variations.[62] As participants learn and grow their skill, you can raise the challenge with each session; even the subtlest adjustments will affect the overall impact of the strokes. Therefore, their advancement isn't just due to the intensity but also their increased understanding of how their bodies are engaged in the water.

TEACHING HIT

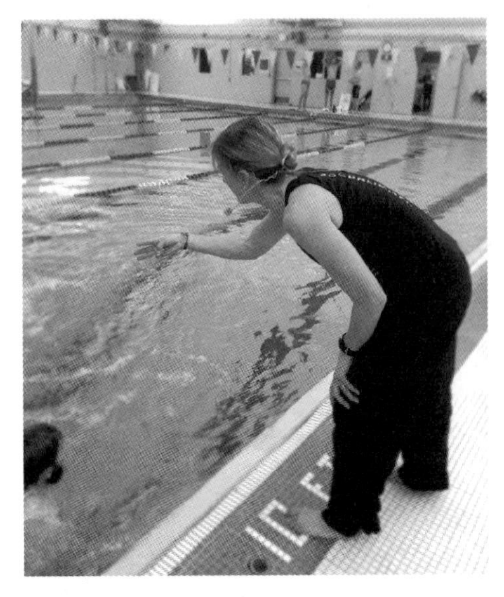

HIT is typically done as a coached workout. It's taught differently from water aerobics, which is conducted similarly to land-based aerobics where the instructor moves through the motions and the participants follow along to the beat of music.

A coach has the additional responsibility of watching the athletes closely and providing structure, corrections, and guidance in order to keep the athletes healthy and training optimally. Therefore, a coach doesn't need to perform along with the participants or wear specific fitness clothing. Clothes that are too baggy or bulky, however, may prevent free movement of limbs for demonstrations and may make it difficult to show the subtler form components. To help you think of this type of instructor, imagine a track or football coach dressed in shorts and a T-shirt, holding a clipboard; they're ready to put the clipboard down at a moment's notice to demonstrate what they may be asking of the athlete.

As mentioned in earlier chapters, the coach demonstrates movements with one leg planted on the pool deck at all times; the actual demonstration occurs with the opposite leg and both arms. This is a safer practice as it keeps the coach/instructor from jumping around on a potentially wet pool deck.

The elevated position of the coach on the deck offers an optimum position to see participants in the water during the workout; it's a vantage point that allows a view from any angle. If you're situated in the water and performing the exercises along with your participants, you can't see their movements or help with form corrections. Therefore, being on the deck will allow you to correct movement patterns and give frequent reminders as well as demonstrations.

NAVIGATING THE WATERS

I've found that teaching in a pool works best when a concerted effort is taken to keep the participants moving in an organized manner and as smoothly as possible in the allotted space. The unusual thing about navigating and maneuvering in water is that it isn't intuitive or familiar. With land-based training, this isn't something that needs to be discussed. Initially with deep water training, this will need to be taught. Management of the participants in the pool is vital to maintaining stroke form and intensities with a large group. This is even more important when there are newer participants.

In addition, navigating the waters is important because participants work at various speeds, traveling faster or slower, and you'll want to avoid bottlenecks (when too many participants end up in the same "space" of water at the same time). With some people traveling faster than others, providing enough room to maneuver allows participants the ability to move around each other. By being aware of this issue and helping to keep the "waters" from becoming crowded or congested, you'll be more likely to give them the workout they desire and bolster satisfaction.

As an analogy, think of cars moving down a heavy traffic-laden road, seamlessly maneuvering around each other as needed. Now, imagine if there weren't any driving laws—cars smash into each other to get to where they want to go...oh wait, isn't that the demolition derby? This isn't what you want to happen in deep water training.

In addition, a group will need an appropriately sized area for an optimum workout. Too many people in close proximity will generate more frustration. For an idea of space parameters, consider a two lane, 25 meter pool of 6 feet in depth (with lane lines taken out). The maximum number would be about 15 to 20 people, but the exact number would depend on the experience level of the group. The higher skilled are better at navigating and can maneuver well with less space per person. Providing sufficient space also allows the group to more comfortably and freely perform the larger range-of-motion exercises with longer reaches and limb extension. Even so, there's still the potential of getting tangled underwater (ask any masters swimmer about the potential of accidentally hitting hands when passing each other).

Even with sufficient room, when the pool space isn't managed, athletes become frustrated. This is something not witnessed much in land-based fitness. I believe the frustration comes from a state of concentrated focus. Athletes are thinking intently about the motions they're performing and, when bumped or contacted, they're almost jolted out of their intense focus. I've seen individuals become very agitated when another participant "invades" their water space or touches them with a hand or foot underwater. If you consider most land-based or shallow-water fitness, participants have clear visibility of their own "space" to perform their exercise without outside forces to contend with.

Those new to deep water training have yet to learn how to perform the strokes correctly, much less grasp water dynamics such as drag and resistance. They likely don't understood what's happening when they move too close to another participant and the effects of the eddy are encountered. By guiding a group to navigate the water, the experienced individuals will feel less frustration (no one's getting in their way; no tangling limbs) and the new participants won't feel pressured as they build proficiency and confidence.

To teach this water navigation, I keep the group moving in a large circle through the pool similar to "circle" swimming for masters swimmers or track practice for runners. I typically work a group in a counterclockwise circle—a method of movement in the water that comes from working on land—shown to me by Sharon Svensson years ago (I spent many hours observing Sharon, as well as Shirley, when honing my skills as an instructor). A clockwise direction can also be used, although to some athletes it can feel unusual, as the counterclockwise movement is the familiar direction to anyone who has ever spent time on a high school or college track. However, this doesn't mean that individuals need to move in a single file line. Quite the contrary. Think of a group moving through the water in the same direction, but with some extra maneuver room to account for the personal eddy currents being generated. By doing so, you'll have participants learn to "navigate" in the water using the spaces that are available.

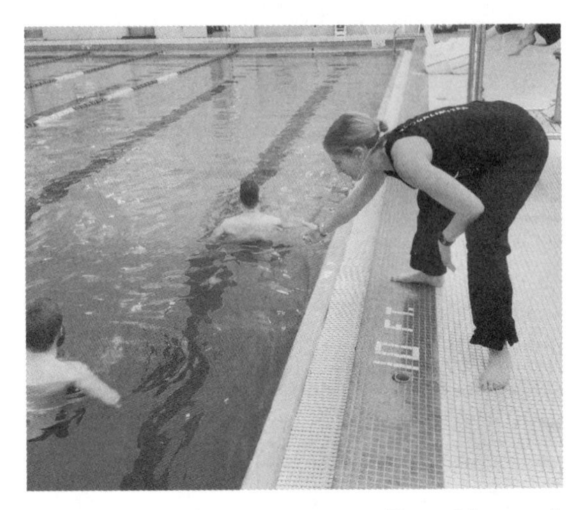

This circling pattern doesn't have to be your method, but I've seen deep water classes in which instructors attempt to teach the same way as a land-based or shallow-water aerobics class where participants have their own allotted "space" to work in for the duration of the class, but I find that class management is challenged. In these instances, the flow of the workouts, not to mention the participants' form, are hampered by the attempt to maintain a specific space in the water. This type of arrangement is also not well suited to the strokes that are purposefully designed for travel in the water.

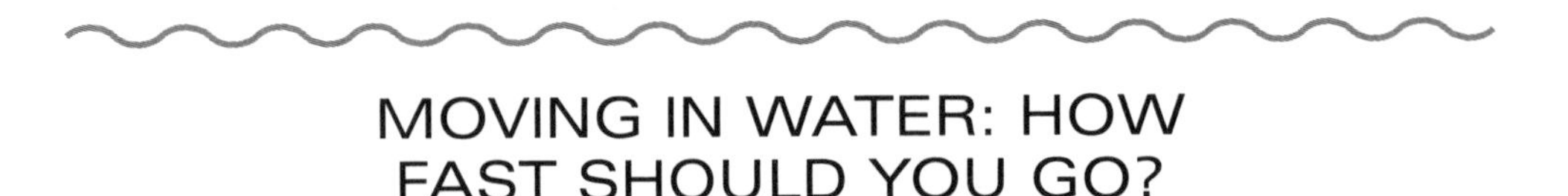

MOVING IN WATER: HOW FAST SHOULD YOU GO?

An important comment to make (and reiterate) to your class is that the speed with which someone moves through the water isn't indicative of how hard they're working. As you recall in Chapters 4 and 5, some people will use a pulling or scooping action that will make them travel faster than others, but this doesn't always mean they're working harder or using the correct form as speed and effort do not always go hand in hand. This reminder will help individuals focus on what they're doing and not try to compete with others by improperly adjusting the stroke.

When traveling, water currents must be considered. They can be compared to running on a windy day; you could have headwinds, tailwinds, and crosswinds that you need to compensate for or accommodate. You don't see them; you feel them. In water, it's the same type of situation.

Therefore, try to suggest that participants start passing when they get to within about four or five feet of another person. Any closer, the eddy current generated by the person being passed will be encountered and act almost like a "tailwind," pulling them together.

I've found that the most challenging group to work with in the water are runners, as they typically want to "pace" and stay a specific and fairly close distance behind others the way they do on land. If they do this in water, they'll be picked up by the current generated by the person in front (i.e., the eddy). As you've learned, the resistance within the eddy is lower and they'll literally be pulled into the person in front of them (part of the frustration I mentioned earlier).

Water current to the side will also need to be considered when passing, just as with a "crosswind" in a car. Individuals will need to maintain at least two to three feet of distance at their sides, depending on the stroke being performed, so they also have enough room for the limb movements. Pass too close, the same "pulling" effect will happen as previously mentioned, and you'll risk limbs tangling underwater. They won't be pushed apart, as some may think.

The essential and continual function of guiding and reminding participants to use the space appropriately is easily done by the coach/trainer who has the best view of the class. Frequent cues to "use your space" or "navigate" will aid in a well-managed and less-frustrated group. It only takes a reminder and a quick glance for participants to maintain the flow.

POSITIVE REINFORCEMENT AND CORRECTING A PARTICIPANT

It's important to invest time to learn the skill of being an instructor, just how you learned your sport. Over the years training, coaching, and conducting group fitness, I've found that my most useful tool has been something many people have heard before: Treat others as you would want to be treated. For me, this means that I'm encouraging my participants when it reinforces proper form or confirms a correct adjustment to form, not randomly just to fill empty air space. When I give feedback regarding someone's movement or form, I'm straightforward and clear with them as to what needs to be changed. Being direct can be better received if done in an honest and nonjudgmental manner. This doesn't mean that I'd make a comment in front of a group, such as "You're doing that wrong." If I were to receive that in front of others, I'd feel embarrassed and discouraged; I wouldn't want to return. But by using an alternative that can mean the same thing but in softer tone and waiting until the participant is the only one within earshot, the correction will be more readily received. Teaching is about supportively guiding, not shoving. A few suggestions for correction: "Try doing it this way..." or "You may 'feel' the exercise more if you...."

TRICK: The technique of providing global corrections can be helpful when working with a large group, typically when a third or more of the group is performing part of the stroke incorrectly. By bringing attention to the incorrect stroke component in a general manner, all participants will concentrate on the specified area. While you describe to the group what you may be seeing, you are also providing the correction that needs to be made. This technique can be quite effective. If a general comment isn't suitable, the opportunity to work one on one privately is also possible by waiting for the individual to travel by your location on the deck and providing your individual cuing more discreetly. This can be done during warm-up or cool-down periods as well. In a standard water fitness class, this opportunity is lost.

MORE HELPFUL TEACHING TIPS

As a coach and educator, I approach workouts with an agenda in mind. I may write out an entire term (since I'm teaching at a university) so that participants progressively advance. This advancement is based on regular and consistent attendance, where workouts can become steadily more challenging, if desired. This strategy of a pre-planned format creates structure for a single workout as well as the entire program spanning several months. It also ensures that the workouts are balanced in timing, effort levels, and targeted muscle groups (as desired).

Reviewing past workouts for potential refinements to the athletes' training based on their responses and their goals is easily done with records of the workouts.

In the fitness arena, you'll hear instructors frequently repeat themselves. We do this to get the attention of the participants because, at any given time, they can be focused inward, be talking to someone else, or be distracted (in water, it can even be the splashing of water around their heads). Therefore, be prepared to give frequent reminders to help maintain focus and control over your class.

In addition, I find it effective to review the following suggestions with the participants while they're just getting into the water and warming up, as you'll have everyone's attention. This ensures that they've all received the same instructions before they begin the actual workout. Some of the reminders suggested are repeated from previous chapters, but they're important enough to state again:

Move at your own pace. Reminders for working at their own pace will help experienced and inexperienced participants alike. The experienced can work harder; the inexperienced can work at an easier effort. This global reminder works for everyone. Deep water interval training can be an intense workout if they choose. Every class can be constructed for various fitness levels, allowing all fitness abilities to participate in one class. An analogy would be a masters swimming workout:

Each lane is divided into various abilities, and the workouts are amended to accommodate all swimmers (experienced may swim 5 x 100 meters; beginners/inexperienced 5 x 50 meters). However, teaching various fitness levels in one group can be challenging for a novice instructor, as you may need to simultaneously direct experienced people to continue working harder and inexperienced to transition to recovery.

Don't do more than you're truly ready to perform. The problem with deep water training is that water can feel so good, supportive, and energizing that inexperienced individuals, or those recently released from rehab, may try to push harder than their bodies are ready to. Frequently remind these individuals to go easier so they can return another day.

Shower before and after getting into the pool. This is helpful for the health of the skin and hair as well as the pool. See page 14 for more information.

Navigate the space: This is my cue for participants to be mindful of where their body is located in the water and to watch where they're traveling. An excellent way to teach them this is to suggest that they not "tailgate," just like when driving a car. Simply go around.

Be aware of "hydro-rage." This is a term I've been using for years when describing what happens when a participant is bumped, splashed, or "cut off" unexpectedly. I've seen participants shoot very angry looks at either me or the person who did the bump/splash/cut-off, almost to say, "Do something." I've witnessed people yell, splash, or even storm out of the pool. It may seem that I'm making this up since it verges on being comical and would seem unbelievable. Amazingly, these examples are true! Understanding and being prepared for these reactions as an instructor is useful in minimizing their occurrence by educating and regularly reminding the group about navigation. My theory is that these types of reactions are due to being startled (as I previously discussed) and not so much related to being physically contacted. In any other fitness format, you can see everyone around you but, in deep water training, you can't see other people's limbs, only their heads. Thus, the "kick" underwater, even if mild, can be almost like an electric jolt.

Minimize talk during the workout. Just like with any other type of group training, try to keep participant talking to a minimum. Because the head and ears are so close to the surface of the pool, sounds in the pool room (such as other coached groups/swim lessons, splashing) seem amplified, making it very difficult to hear an instructor, even when using a microphone. Now, imagine adding conversations among participants. This doesn't mean that deep water training can't be social—introduce fun and conversation at the appropriate times by planning them into your workout.

Be careful when exiting the pool. For some individuals who haven't had adequate recovery, exiting the pool can have an effect of lowering blood pressure, which is noticed by a participant in the guise of dizziness, lightheadedness, and weakness. I don't see it often, but it does occasionally occur. If this happens, having the participant sit or even lie down can help with symptoms until the blood pressure rises again. If the symptoms are severe, have the participant lie down on the floor and prop the legs up on a chair or bench so that they're higher than the heart. Wait for symptoms to subside.

MISCELLANEOUS TIDBITS FOR POOL-BASED INSTRUCTION

The following are some basic tips with a few of my own twists that I've used over the years. Many can also be found in other water training books. I feel they're important enough to mention:

BELT FIT

A belt is usually worn below the navel, cinched down snugly to keep it from pressing down (squeezing) on the ribcage, making it difficult to breathe. The flotation portion goes around the waist and against the back. Plan on teaching a first-time participant how to use the belt and how to tighten it before getting into the pool. Have participants put the belt on when they're still on dry deck. Then, when they think it's tight, show them how to give the belt a sharp and quick tug. The quick tug will cinch the belt down. It may feel tight on deck but once submerged underwater, the participant's body will "decrease in size" due to the hydrostatic pressure. If the belt is too tight, they can easily let a bit of the tension out as needed. If the belt isn't tight enough, it will ride up the waist and the flotation will rub on the inner arms in many of the movements. Note that individuals with a higher body-fat content may not need a belt at all because their bodies are buoyant enough to keep their chins above the water; allow them to chose if they want to wear one or not.

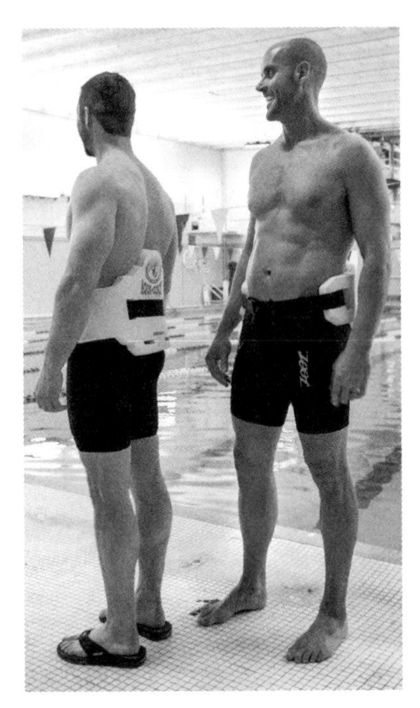

Note: When working with pregnant participants, situate the belt so that it's not "on" the belly; possibly run it under the belly. In some cases, I've had participants wear it above their belly, but be prepared for the belt to ride up under the armpits. A belt that high can affect upper-body movement and has the potential of chafing under the arms.

STAY ON THE DRY DECK

The view from the deck allows you to maximize your effectiveness as an instructor and carry out the training instructions included in this book. A dry deck is also important for your own personal safety. As deep water training doesn't lend itself to standing in one spot, I don't use the "teaching mat" that many aqua aerobics instructors use. Instead, I walk around the pool deck, being mindful of puddles and the potential for slipping. I've even dried puddles prior to working on a pool deck.

GOOD VISION

If you're working with large groups, potentially taking up four or even five pool lanes, you'll need to view people through the water at a distance. You'll need to have the ability to see well up to 30 feet. Bodies are distorted by the movement of water; therefore, good vision and ease of deck mobility is important. Without it, you're not able to coach adequately.

MUSIC VS. NO MUSIC

Playing music with a deep water workout is a personal preference. I've worked with both with equal results. Incorporating background music allows participants to use it for motivation. Over the years, though, I've had some groups find the music distracting, as deep water training takes immense focus for many people, especially those new to the workout. Many coached workouts don't have music, so if you don't use music, your role becomes even more important as a motivator. If music is desired for sets, then choreographing the drills would be necessary (e.g., quicker music to faster-paced drills). However, watch for participants sacrificing form in their attempt to stay with the beat.

USE A MICROPHONE

I've taught for many years and realized that my voice is my most important tool. Depending on the acoustics of the space, the noise level from other people, and water noise, your voice can become easily strained. You'll need to project over all sounds around a pool deck, so respect and protect your valuable asset. Purchase a microphone (mic) and use it every time, whether you think you need it or not. Prices vary, but a simple portable system with a detached mic/battery pack can cost as little as $50.

ACQUIRE A LARGE CLOCK OR TIMER

A timepiece is important for timing your sets. I use my watch in every class because exercise/recovery ratios are very specific with interval training. However, having a large clock with a second hand placed where participants can see is helpful if working with cadence as well as allows participants to know where they're at in a set.

GET CERTIFIED

As I've stated, this book can help you participate in deep water interval training as a participant or an instructor. But to maximize your effectiveness as a facilitator, I recommend certification in coaching, personal training, and/or group fitness.

PRACTICE BEFORE YOU TEACH

If you're stepping into the role of an instructor, practice how you'll teach and instruct each move before walking onto that pool deck. The participants are counting on you to be their guide, and you'll need to be able to stand on the pool deck in full view, call out a move, and properly demonstrate it. Your credibility will soar if you can do that. In addition, coming into deep water interval training without mastering the exercises yourself isn't recommended. You need to know what the movements will feel like in order to verbally cue them. Plan on practicing the exercises with a friend to work on form or taking a deep water training workshop.

CHARISMA AND PASSION

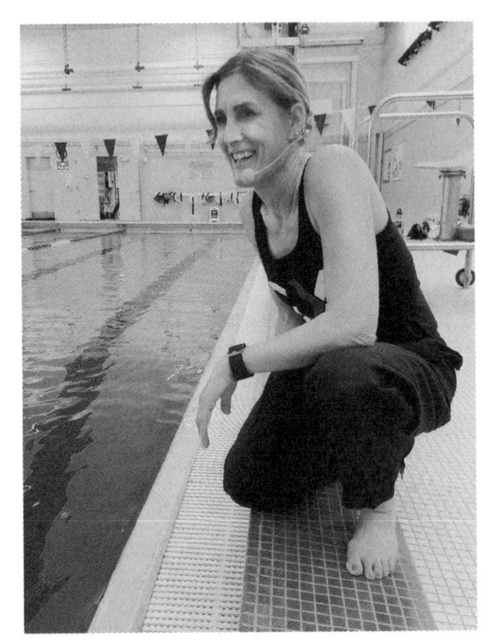

Having charisma, passion, and the desire to teach will do wonders for your career. The group will respond to someone who's engaged in what they're asking others to do. This means that you're energetic, but you don't necessarily need to be a cheerleader (anyone who has watched me teach would tell you that I'm not!). Other highly beneficial qualities that can be developed over time are a sense of ease being in front of a group of people, an attention to detail (such as with timing, form, and function), a sense of confidence when giving directions and correcting individuals, and comfort in challenging them to push outside of their comfort zones.

HAVE FUN

I enjoy what I do and have fun every time even after 20-plus years. Yes, FUN. If you don't enjoy working with people, then working with groups is probably not the right fit. In all my years of teaching and coaching (sometimes 20 hours a week), I've yet to experience teaching a group without enjoying it!

Teaching, for me, has been a large part of my life. It has made me laugh to the point of tears and it has brought many amazing and wonderful people, including my husband, into my life. I enjoy every minute of working with people and helping them improve their lives through fitness. This, to me, has been one of the greatest gifts I've given others. Yet, at the same time, it's one of the greatest gifts I've given myself.

We hope this book inspires you to work in the water, and train and coach people on a platform that can allow people to work hard and train their entire lives, living to their full, athletic potential. We also hope that after reading this book, you're one more member of the growing community that believes that deep water training is the key to unlock the fitness potential of many and can help others continue to achieve, as well as enhance, the athleticism they value and to which they have grown accustomed.

Glossary

Aerobic effort: This is an effort that increases the heart rate to a level that can be maintained for an extended period of time. At this level, the body is capable of replenishing oxygen usage. This aerobic effort is most effective for fat-burning and ideal for endurance training.

Anaerobic effort: This is a short-lasting, high-intensity effort that increases the heart rate to a level that cannot be sustained for an extended period of time. At this level, the body is not capable of meeting the oxygen demands of the effort and relies on limited energy sources stored within the muscles. This is an ideal effort used in interval training, also known as threshold work. Anaerobic training also improves aerobic function and overall fitness.

Back position: The location of a limb when it is behind the body.

Borg Rating of Perceived Exertion (Borg scale): This rating method, developed by Gunnar Borg, uses a numbering system to gauge the intensity level of physical activity. Also known as the RPE (rate of perceived exertion) scale.

Breakout stroke (BOS): A stroke where you increase effort for a determined target time, after which point you return to a steady state.

Buoyancy: This is the "lifting" effect, or the upward force a body experiences in water; it's the force that makes the body float.

Cadence: The number of cycles a leg moves in a minute. Also known as turnover.

Catch: The start of the stroke, when the hand or leg begins the power phase.

Center of gravity (CG): The point at which your weight is evenly distributed in all directions when you're on land, making you feel stable and balanced. This stability point is located around the hips/pelvis region.

Center of buoyancy (CB): Similar to the center of gravity (CG) on land, the center of buoyancy (CB) in water is the balance point that's located closer to the chest.

Closed kinetic chain: An exercise with a closed kinetic chain is performed with a hand or foot fixed and in contact with an immovable object, most often the ground. A squat is an example of a lower-limb exercise with a closed kinetic chain.

Core: All the muscles of the central portion of the body from the neck to the hips. This includes the gluteals, abdominals, rib and chest muscles, spinal muscles (from the neck to the lower back), and scapular muscles.

Density: Technically, density is the mass-per-unit volume or how compact or solid something is. In water, density can be felt as "thickness."

Dorsiflexion: The upward ankle motion used to move the foot or toes toward the shin.

Drag: The force that acts to oppose the body's movement. Drag is felt as resistance to motion.

Drive: The powerful motion of the limbs during a stroke.

Extension: A position created by straightening a joint (increasing the joint angle associated between two bones).

Flexion: A position created by bending a joint (decreasing the joint angle associated between two bones).

Follow-through: The process of completing a limb movement.

Forward position: The location of a limb when it is in front of the body.

Frontal plane: An imaginary vertical line that divides the body into two portions, a back and front. Also known as the coronal plane.

Gravity: The force that works to pull objects, including the body, toward the ground.

Hitching: A form issue that's typically seen in the Water Run when the rear/hips incorrectly shift up and back, rather than stay elongated and in line with the spine.

Horizontal plane: An imaginary horizontal line that divides the body into an upper and lower section, the midpoint being at about the navel. Also known as the transverse plane.

Hydro interval training (HIT): An interval-based, full-body workout where all exercises are performed in deep water without a fixed surface to stabilize the body.

Hydrostatic pressure (HP): The pressure of the weight of the water that envelopes the body. The deeper a person is submerged, the more HP exerts its force on the body.

Interval training: A type of training that involves variable durations and intensities, typically working up to maximum efforts, with the ultimate purpose to improve overall endurance. In water, this also results in additional strength gains due to the increased resistance.

Jabbing: A description of when legs drive away from and back toward the body without any sweeping or scooping motion, such as when correctly performing the High Knee or Straight-Shot Punch.

Kinesthetic awareness: The awareness or ability to sense where your body is within space. Also known as body awareness.

Lower limbs: The legs.

Maximum effort: The effort at the top range of a person's ability to perform a given workout set.

Midline: An imaginary vertical line on the body that divides the right and left sides equally. Also known as the median or midsagittal plane.

Open kinetic chain: An exercise where the hands and feet move freely. All deep water strokes are examples of exercises with open kinetic chains.

Overreaching: Extending the limbs farther than is intended based on the stroke descriptions.

Overrotate: This is a result of an upper and/or lower limb overreaching forward and backward, causing a rotational misalignment not intended for the specific stroke. With the arm, it's seen as the upper torso excessively rotating forward or backward; with the leg, it's seen as the hip or the pelvis excessively rotating forward or backward.

Plantarflexion: The downward ankle motion used to move the foot or toes away from the shin; pointing the toes.

Power phase: The stage of the stroke where you apply the most effort or force. Greater effort increases the intensity of the motion. A stroke's power phase follows the catch.

Progressive exercise: Exercise that starts at an easy pace then gradually increases speed or effort.

Pull: During the stroke, the powerful motion of the limbs toward the body.

Range of motion (ROM): ROM is the degree of motion of the limbs while performing a stroke. It is not used here in the same context as some health professionals do for specific joint motion. ROM varies for each person.

Repetition (rep): The number of times a given exercise is to be performed; typically prescribed in a "set."

Recovery: There are two types of recovery: movement and physiological. In movement, this is seen as the return of a limb to the start of a power phase (also referred to as recovery phase). In the physiological context, it's used to describe three situations: 1) the time between interval sets, 2) the time at the end of a workout routine (aka a cool-down), and 3) part of a weekly/monthly or even yearly training pattern.

Rotation: The turning motion (pivot) of the body around a joint axis. An example is moving a hand from a palm facing down to a palm facing up.

Sagittal plane: An imaginary vertical line that divides the body into right and left sides at any point on the body, creating uneven left and right sections. A midsagittal (midline) plane divides the sides equally.

Scooping: This refers to when you rigidly curve or cup a hand/foot that should be held straight, which causes you to scoop water when the limb is in motion. When this is done with the hand, it appears as if you are trying to "dig" at the water.

Sculling: A technique to hold yourself above the water by using outstretched arms to make sweeping figure-eight motions along the plane of the water's surface.

Set: The number of times, or cycles, you repeat a series of repetitions.

Steady-state exercise: Exercise that maintains a constant speed or effort over the duration of the set.

Target heart rate: This is the aerobic range you should exercise in for the best workout results; it's typically 55 to 85% of your maximum heart rate. A safe aquatic target heart rate is 20 to 30% less than your land-based one.

Transverse plane: *See* Horizontal plane.

T-rexing: A shortened upper limb movement seen when the arms do not go through a full range of motion, usually stopping about six inches before the hips rather than just slightly beyond the hips.

Turbulence: Agitated water movement created by the body's movement in water.

Upper limbs: The arms.

Viscosity: The "thickness" of a fluid, experienced as the resistance to motion when moving through the water.

Notes

1. Charles L. Lowman et al., *Technique of Underwater Gymnastics: A Study in Practical Application* (Los Angeles, CA: American Publications, 1937): 6.

2. Kevin E. Wilk and David M. Joyner, *Use of Aquatics in Orthopedics and Sports Medicine Rehabilitation and Physical Conditioning* (Therofare, NJ: Slack Incorporated, 2014): 3.

3. Charles L. Lowman et al., *Technique of Underwater Gymnastics: A Study in Practical Application* (Los Angeles, CA: American Publications, 1937): 66.

4. Steve Tarpinian and Brian Awbrey, *Water Workouts: A Guide to Fitness, Training, and Performance Enhancement in the Water* (New York: Lyons Press, 1997): 3, 58, 105, 109.

5. P. D. Pantoja et al., "Effect of Resistive Exercise on Muscle Damage in Water and on Land," *Journal of Strength and Conditioning Research* 23 (May 2009): 1051.

6. Orna A. Donoghue et al., "Impact Forces of Plyometric Exercises Performed on Land and in Water," *Sports Health* 3, no. 3 (May 2011): 309.

7. A. H. Ploeg et al., "The Effects of High Volume Aquatic Plyometric Training on Vertical Jump, Muscle Power, and Torque," *International Journal of Aquatic Research and Education* 4, no. 1 (2010): 40.

8. A. H. Ploeg et al., "The Effects of High Volume Aquatic Plyometric Training on Vertical Jump, Muscle Power, and Torque," *International Journal of Aquatic Research and Education* 4, no. 1 (2010): 39–40.

9. David Brennan, "Deep Water Running," *Aquarunning*, Orthopedic Hospital of Oklahoma, Houston International Running Center (2003): 1.

10. Michael Moon, *Deep Water Exercise for High Performance Sport* (Victoria, BC: Trafford Publishing, 2009): 18.

11. David Brennan, "Deep Water Running," *Aquarunning*, Orthopedic Hospital of Oklahoma, Houston International Running Center (2003): 1.

12. Joel Friel, *Fast after 50: How to Race Strong for the Rest of Your Life* (Boulder, Colorado: VeloPress, 2015).

13. Cristine Lima Alberton et al., "Kinesiological Analysis of Stationary Running Performed in Aquatic and Dry Land Environments," *Journal of Human Kinetics* 49 (2015): 5.

14. Kevin E. Wilk and David M. Joyner, *Use of Aquatics in Orthopedics and Sports Medicine Rehabilitation and Physical Conditioning* (Therofare, NJ: Slack Incorporated, 2014): 7.

15. ACSM Issues New Recommendations on Quantity and Quality of Exercise," American College of Sports Medicine, accessed May 2016, http://www.acsm.org/about-acsm/media-room/news-releases/2011/08/01/acsm-issues-new-recommendations-on-quantity-and-quality-of-exercise.

16. Mimi Rodriquez Adami, *Aqua Fitness: The Low-Impact Total Body Fitness Workout* (New York: DK Publishing, 2002): 9.

17. Karl Knopf, *Make the Pool Your Gym: No-Impact Water Workouts for Getting Fit, Building Strength and Rehabbing from Injury* (Berkeley, CA: Ulysses Press, 2012): 10.

18. M. R. Assis et al., "Controlled Trial of Deep Water Running: Clinical Effectiveness of Aquatic Exercise to Treat Fibromyalgia," *American College of Rheumatology* 55, no. 1 (2006): 58.

19. Bruce Becker, "Aquatic Therapy: Scientific Foundations and Clinical Rehabilitation Applications," *American Academy of Physical Medicine and Rehabilitation* 1 (2009): 863.

20. David Brennan, "Deep Water Running," *Aquarunning*, Orthopedic Hospital of Oklahoma, Houston International Running Center, (2003): 2.

21. Kevin E. Wilk and David M. Joyner, *Use of Aquatics in Orthopedics and Sports Medicine Rehabilitation and Physical Conditioning* (Thorofare, NJ: Slack Incorporated, 2014): 5–6.

22. Kevin E. Wilk and David M. Joyner, *Use of Aquatics in Orthopedics and Sports Medicine Rehabilitation and Physical Conditioning* (Thorofare, NJ: Slack Incorporated, 2014): 8–9.

23. Michael Moon, *Deep Water Exercise for High Performance Sport* (Victoria, BC: Trafford Publishing, 2009): 21.

24. Bruce Becker, "Aquatic Therapy: Scientific Foundations and Clinical Rehabilitation Applications," *American Academy of Physical Medicine and Rehabilitation* 1 (2009): 860.

25. Anthony S. Burns and Tamara D. Lauder, "Deep Water Running: An Effective Non-Weightbearing Exercise for the Maintenance of Land-Based Running Performance." *Military Medicine* 166, no. 3 (March 2001): 253.

26. Anthony S. Burns and Tamara D. Lauder, "Deep Water Running: An Effective Non-Weightbearing Exercise for the Maintenance of Land-Based Running Performance." *Military Medicine* 166 no. 3 (March 2001): 253.

27. Bruce Becker, "Aquatic Therapy: Scientific Foundations and Clinical Rehabilitation Applications," *American Academy of Physical Medicine and Rehabilitation* 1 (2009): 860.

28. Aquatic Exercise Association, *Aquatic Fitness Professional Manual: The Definitive Resource for AEA Certification and All-In-One Reference Guide*, 6th ed., (Champaign, IL: Human Kinetics, 2010): 186.

29. Aquatic Exercise Association, *Aquatic Fitness Professional Manual: The Definitive Resource for AEA Certification and All-In-One Reference Guide*, 6th ed., (Champaign, IL: Human Kinetics, 2010): 189–190.

30. Aquatic Exercise Association, *Aquatic Fitness Professional Manual: The Definitive Resource for AEA Certification and All-In-One Reference Guide*, 6th ed., (Champaign, IL: Human Kinetics, 2010): 100–101.

31. A. H. Ploeg et al., "The Effects of High Volume Aquatic Plyometric Training on Vertical Jump, Muscle Power, and Torque," *International Journal of Aquatic Research and Education* 4, no. 1 (2010): 40.

32. Mimi Rodriquez Adami, *Aqua Fitness: The Low-Impact Total Body Fitness Workout* (New York: DK Publishing, 2002): 10.

33. Kevin E. Wilk and David M. Joyner, *Use of Aquatics in Orthopedics and Sports Medicine Rehabilitation and Physical Conditioning* (Thorofare, NJ: Slack Incorporated, 2014): 93.

34. A. H. Ploeg et al., "The Effects of High Volume Aquatic Plyometric Training on Vertical Jump, Muscle Power, and Torque," *International Journal of Aquatic Research and Education* 4, no. 1 (2010): 40.

35. Kevin E. Wilk and David M. Joyner, *Use of Aquatics in Orthopedics and Sports Medicine Rehabilitation and Physical Conditioning* (Thorofare, NJ: Slack Incorporated, 2014): 21.

36. Gregory G. Haff, "Aquatic Cross Training for Athletes: Part 1," *Strength & Conditioning Journal* 30, no. 2 (2008).

37. Gregory G. Haff, "Aquatic Cross Training for Athletes: Part 2," *Strength & Conditioning Journal* 30, no. 3 (2008): 68.

38. Karl Knopf, *Make the Pool Your Gym: No-Impact Water Workouts for Getting Fit, Building Strength and Rehabbing from Injury* (Berkeley, CA: Ulysses Press, 2012): 15.

39. Aquatic Exercise Association, *Aquatic Fitness Professional Manual: The Definitive Resource for AEA Certification and All-In-One Reference Guide*, 6th ed., (Champaign, IL: Human Kinetics, 2010): 85–86.

40. Adapted from *Use of Aquatics in Orthopedics and Sports Medicine* by Kevin E. Wilk and David M. Joyner.

41. Aquatic Exercise Association, *Aquatic Fitness Professional Manual: The Definitive Resource for AEA Certification and All-In-One Reference Guide*, 6th ed., (Champaign, IL: Human Kinetics, 2010): 85.

42. Kevin E. Wilk and David M. Joyner, *Use of Aquatics in Orthopedics and Sports Medicine Rehabilitation and Physical Conditioning* (Thorofare, NJ: Slack Incorporated, 2014): 6.

43. Gregory G. Haff, "Aquatic Cross Training for Athletes: Part 1," *Strength & Conditioning Journal* 30, no. 2 (2008): 18.

44. Maria Hutsick, "Hydro Power, Training & Conditioning," last modified January 29, 2015, accessed June 2016, http://training-conditioning.com/2007/03/09/hydro_power/index.php.

45. Maria Hutsick, "Hydro Power, Training & Conditioning," last modified January 29, 2015, accessed June 2016, http://training-conditioning.com/2007/03/09/hydro_power/index.php.

46. Maria Hutsick, "Hydro Power, Training & Conditioning," last modified January 29, 2015, accessed June 2016, http://training-conditioning.com/2007/03/09/hydro_power/index.php.

47. T. Reichert et al., "Continuous and interval training programs using deep water running improves functional fitness and blood pressure in older adults," *Age* 38, no. 1 (2016): 5.

48. MaryBeth Pappas Baun, *Fantastic Water Workouts: Proven Exercises and Routines for Toning, Fitness, and Health*, 2nd ed., (Champaign, IL: Human Kinetics, 2008): 11.

49. Aquatic Exercise Association, *Aquatic Fitness Professional Manual: The Definitive Resource for AEA Certification and All-In-One Reference Guide*, 6th ed., (Champaign, IL: Human Kinetics, 2010): 6–8.

50. Aquatic Exercise Association, *Aquatic Fitness Professional Manual: The Definitive Resource for AEA Certification and All-In-One Reference Guide*, 6th ed., (Champaign, IL: Human Kinetics, 2010): 6–7.

51. Aquatic Exercise Association, *Aquatic Fitness Professional Manual: The Definitive Resource for AEA Certification and All-In-One Reference Guide*, 6th ed., (Champaign, IL: Human Kinetics, 2010): 6.

52. Kevin E. Wilk and David M. Joyner, *Use of Aquatics in Orthopedics and Sports Medicine Rehabilitation and Physical Conditioning* (Thorofare, NJ: Slack Incorporated, 2014): 58.

53. David Brennan, "Deep Water Running," *Aquarunning*, Orthopedic Hospital of Oklahoma, Houston International Running Center (2003): 3.

54. Kevin E. Wilk and David M. Joyner, *Use of Aquatics in Orthopedics and Sports Medicine Rehabilitation and Physical Conditioning* (Thorofare, NJ: Slack Incorporated, 2014): 57–58.

55. MaryBeth Pappas Baun, *Fantastic Water Workouts: Proven Exercises and Routines for Toning, Fitness, and Health*, 2nd ed., (Champaign, IL: Human Kinetics, 2008): 11.

56. Aquatic Exercise Association, *Aquatic Fitness Professional Manual: The Definitive Resource for AEA Certification and All-In-One Reference Guide*, 6th ed., (Champaign, IL: Human Kinetics, 2010): 100–101.

57. Aquatic Exercise Association, *Aquatic Fitness Professional Manual: The Definitive Resource for AEA Certification and All-In-One Reference Guide*, 6th ed., (Champaign, IL: Human Kinetics, 2010): 197.

58. David Brennan, "Deep Water Running," *Aquarunning*, Orthopedic Hospital of Oklahoma, Houston International Running Center (2003): 3.

59. David Brennan, "Deep Water Running," *Aquarunning*, Orthopedic Hospital of Oklahoma, Houston International Running Center (2003): 3.

60. Azar Nafisi, *Reading Lolita in Tehran: A Memoir in Books* (New York: Random House, 2003): 8.

61. Marietta Mehanni, "Deeply Moving," *Marietta Mehanni*, accessed March 2017, www.mariettamehanni.com/articles/aqua/109-deeply-moving

62. Christine Alexander, *Water Fitness Lesson Plans and Choreography: 72 Lesson Plans and 576 Activities for Shallow and Deep Water* (Champaign, IL: Human Kinetics, 2011): 5–9.

References

"ACSM Issues New Recommendations on Quantity and Quality of Exercise." *American College of Sports Medicine.* Last modified August 1, 2011. Accessed June 2016. www.acsm.org/about-acsm/media-room/news-releases/2011/08/01/acsm-issues-new-recommendations-on-quantity-and-quality-of-exercise.

Adami, Mimi Rodriguez. *Aqua Fitness: The Low-Impact Total Body Fitness Workout.* New York: DK Publishing, 2002.

Alberton, C. L., S. S. Pinto, N. A. da Silva Azenha, E. L. Cadore, M. P. Tartaruga, B. Brasil, and L. F. M. Kruel. "Kinesiological Analysis of Stationary Running Performed in Aquatic and Dryland Environments." *Journal of Human Kinetics* 49 (2015): 5–14.

Alexander, Christine. *Water Fitness Lesson Plans and Choreography: 72 Lesson Plans and 576 Activities for Shallow and Deep Water.* Champaign, IL: Human Kinetics, 2011.

Aquatic Exercise Association (AEA). *Aquatic Fitness Professional Manual: The Definitive Resource for AEA Certification and All-in-One Reference Guide.* 6th ed. Champaign, IL: Human Kinetics, 2010.

Assis, M. R., Silva, L. E., Alves, A. M. B., Pessanha, A. P., Valim, V., Feldman, D., de Barros Neto, T. L. and Natour, J. "A Randomized Controlled Trial of Deep Water Running: Clinical Effectiveness of Aquatic Exercise to Treat Fibromyalgia." *American College of Rheumatology* 55, no. 1 (2006): 57–65.

Baun, MaryBeth Pappas. *Fantastic Water Workouts: Proven Exercises and Routines for Toning, Fitness, and Health.* 2nd ed. Champaign, IL: Human Kinetics, 2008.

Becker, Bruce. "Aquatic Therapy: Scientific Foundations and Clinical Rehabilitation Applications." *American Academy of Physical Medicine and Rehabilitation* 1 (2009), 859–872. http://aquaticdoc.com/Aquaticdoc.com/Publications_files/Aquatic%20Therapy-%20Scientific%20Aspects.pdf.

Borreli, Lizette. *Medical Daily: How Water Aerobics Help You Stay Fit and Live Longer.* Last modified June 25, 2013. www.medicaldaily.com/how-water-aerobics-help-you-stay-fit-and-live-longer-247119.

Brennan, David. "Deep Water Running." *Aquarunning.* Orthopedic Hospital of Oklahoma: Oklahoma Human Performance Center. Houston International Running Center (2003).

Brody, Lori Thein, and Paula Richley Geigle. *Aquatic Exercise for Rehabilitation and Training.* Champaign, IL: Human Kinetics, 2009.

Burns, Anthony S., and Tamara Lauder. "Deep Water Running: An Effective Non-Weightbearing Exercise for the Maintenance of Land-Based Running Performance." *Military Medicine* 166, no. 3 (2001): 253–258.

Cespedes, Andrea. "Water Aerobics Benefits." Last modified August 16, 2013. www.livestrong.com/article/133611-water-aerobics-benefits/.

Chewning, June. "Understanding Aquatic Heart Rate Deductions." *Fitness Learning Systems.* Accessed June 2016. www.fitnesslearningsystems.com/author_articles/chewning_aquatic_heart_rate_deductions.pdf.

Chewning, J. M., P. S. Krist, and P. A. Poli de Figueiredo. "Monitoring Your Aquatic Heart Rate: Increasing Accuracy with the Kruel Aquatic Adaptation." Aquatic Exercise Association Research Committee. Project conducted May 2008–July 2009. Accessed June 2016. www.aeawave.com/Portals/2/Research/Kruel_research.pdf

Cuesta-Vargas, A. I., J. Buchan, and M. Arroyo-Morales. "A Multimodal Physiotherapy Program Plus Deep Water Running for Improving Cancer-Related Fatigue and Quality of Life in Breast Cancer Survivors." *European Journal of Cancer Care* 23 (2013): 15–21.

Cuesta-Vargas, A. I., N. Adams, J. A. Salazar, A. Belles, S. Hazanas, and M. Arroyo-Morales. "Deep Water Running and General Practice in Primary Care for Non-Specific Low Back Pain Versus General Practice Alone: Randomized Controlled Trial." *Clinical Rheumatology* 31 (2012): 1073–1078.

Donoghue, Orna A., Hirofumi Shimojo, and Hideki Takagi. "Impact Forces of Plyometric Exercises Performed on Land and in Water." *Sports Health* 3, no. 3 (May 2011): 303–309.

Dreyer, Danny, and Katherine Dreyer. *Chi Running: A Revolutionary Approach to Effortless, Injury-Free Running.* New York: Fireside, Simon & Schuster, 2009.

Friel, Joel. *Fast after Fifty: How to Race Strong for the Rest of Your Life.* Boulder, CO: Velo Press, 2015.

Haff, Gregory G. "Aquatic Cross Training for Athletes: Part 1." *National Strength and Conditioning Association* 30, no. 2 (2008): 18–26.

Haff, Gregory G. "Aquatic Cross Training for Athletes: Part 2." *National Strength and Conditioning Association* 30, no. 3 (2008): 67–73.

Hutsick, Maria. "Hydro Power." *Training & Conditioning.* Last modified January 29, 2015. http://training-conditioning.com/2007/03/09/hydro_power/index.php.

Kantz, A. C., R. S. Delevatti, T. Reichert, G. V. Liedtke, R. Ferrari, B. P. Almada, S. S. Pinto, C. L. Alberton, and L. F. M. Kruel. "Effects of Two Deep Water Training Programs on Cardiorespiratory and Muscular Strength Responses in Older Adults." *Experimental Gerontology* 64 (2015): 55–61.

Killgore, G. L., S. C. Coste, S. E. O'Meara, and C. J. Konnecke. "A Comparison of the Physiological Exercise Intensity Differences Between Shod and Barefoot Submaximal Deep-Water Running at the Same Cadence." *Journal of Strength & Conditioning* 12 (2010): 3302–12.

Kravitz, L., and J. J. Mayo. "The Physiological Effects of Aquatic Exercise: A Brief Review." The University of New Mexico. Last modified 1997. Accessed June 2016. www.unm.edu/~lkravitz/Article%20folder/aqua.html.

Lowman, C. L., S. G. Roen, R. Aust, and H. G. Paull. *Technique of Underwater Gymnastic: A Study in Practical Application.* Los Angeles: American Publications, 1937.

Mackenzie, Brian, and Glen Cordoza. *Power Speed Endurance: A Skill-Based Approach to Endurance Training.* Las Vegas: Victory Belt Publishing, 2012.

Martel, G. F., M. L. Harmer, J. M. Logan, and C. B. Parker. "Aquatic Plyometric Training Increases Vertical Jump in Female Volleyball Players." *Medicine & Science in Sports & Exercise* 37, no. 10 (October 2005): 1814–1819.

McHale, Mary E. R. "Water Quality: Salinity vs. Chloride." *CBEN Summer Academy*. Rice University. Last modified February 27, 2007. Accessed August 2, 2016. Rice University. www.ruf.rice.edu/~c-bensa/Salinity.

Mehanni, Marietta. "Deeply Moving." *Marietta Mehanni*. Accessed March 2017. www.mariettame-hanni.com/articles/aqua/109-deeply-moving.

Miller, M. G., C. C. Cheatham, A. R. Porter, M. D. Ricard, D. Hennigar, and D. C. Berry. "Chest- and Waist-Deep Aquatic Plyometric Training and Average Force, Power, and Vertical-Jump Performance." *International Journal of Aquatic Research and Education* 1 (2007): 145–155.

Moon, Michael. *Deep Water Exercise for High Performance Sport: A Training Manual for Athletes and Coaches*. Victoria, BC: Trafford Publishing, 2009.

Nafisi, Azar. *Reading Lolita in Tehran: A Memoir in Books*. New York: Random House, 2003.

Pantoja, P. D., C. L. Alberton, C. Pilla, A. P. Vendrusculo, and L. F. Kruel. "Effect of Resistive Exercise on Muscle Damage in Water and on Land." *Journal of Strength and Conditioning Research* 23, no. 3 (May 2009): 1051–1054.

Pinto, S. S., C. L. Alberton, P. Zaffari, E. L. Cadore, A. C. Kanitz, G. V. Liedtke, M. P. Tartaruga, and L. F. M. Kruel. "Rating of Perceived Exertion and Physiological Responses in Water-Based Exercise." *Journal of Human Kinetics* 49 (2015): 99–108.

Pinto, S. S., E. L. Cadore, C. L. Alberton, E. M. Silva, A. C. Kanitz, M. P. Tartaruga, and L. F. M. Kruel. "Cardiorespiratory and Neuromuscular Responses during Water Aerobics Exercise Performed with and without Equipment." *International Journal of Sports Medicine* 32 (2011): 916–923.

Ploeg, A. H., M. G. Miller, W. R. Holcomb, J. O'Donoghue, D. Berry, and T. J. Dibbet. "The Effects of High Volume Aquatic Plyometric Training on Vertical Jump, Muscle Power, and Torque." *International Journal of Aquatic Research and Education* 4 (2010): 39–48.

Reichert, T., A. C. Kanitz, R. S. Delevatti, N. C. Bagatini, B. M. Barroso, and L. F. M. Kruel. "Continuous and Interval Training Programs Using Deep Water Running Improves Functional Fitness and Blood Pressure in the Older Adults." *AGE: Journal of the American Aging Association* 38 (2016): 20.

Robinson, L. E., S. T. Devor, M. A. Merrick, and J. Buckworth. "The Effects of Land vs. Aquatic Plyometrics on Power, Torque, Velocity, and Muscle Soreness in Women." *The Journal of Strength and Conditioning Research* 18, no. 1 (February 2004): 84–91.

Ruby, Abby. "A New Kind of Brick: Try Aquajogging to Boost Your Run." ACTIVE.com. Last modified 2017. Accessed June 2016. www.active.com/triathlon/articles/a-new-kind-of-brick-try-aquajogging-to-boost-your-run.

Schulke, Flip. *Witness to Our Times: My Life as a Photojournalist*. Chicago: Cricket Books, 2003.

Svinicki, Marilla, and Wilbert J. McKeachie. *Teaching Tips: Strategies, Research, and Theory for College and University Teachers*. 13th ed. Belmont, CA: Wadsworth Publishing Company, 2011.

Tarpinian, Steve and Brian Awbrey. *Water Workouts: A Guide to Fitness, Training, and Performance Enhancement in the Water*. New York: Lyons & Burford, 1997.

Wilk, K. E., and D. M. Joyner. *The Use of Aquatics in Orthopedics and Sports Medicine Rehabilitation and Physical Conditioning*. Thorofare, NJ: Slack Incorporated, 2014.

Index

Acknowledgments

This book has been a quest—a journey, so to speak—cultivated by our lives, passions, experiences, friends, patients, and clients. It has culminated in the words you've read and wouldn't have been possible without the harmonious synchronization of every aspect of this project.

We know *Deep End of the Pool Workouts* wouldn't have materialized without the following people who helped make it happen: Bridget Thoreson of Ulysses Press, who received an unsolicited manuscript and, instead of turning it away with a polite "Thank you for submitting, however...." note, opened the package and read the proposal; Claire Chun, our brilliant editor, who took our words, thoughts, and stories and made them into a book; Shirley Archer, JD, Sharon Svensson, DC, and Kristina Irvin, DC, who guided Melis into a world of water and endurance training and encouraged her growth as a person and coach; Dr. Robert Wilson, who channeled our thoughts of writing a book into the actual process of writing one; our photographers Dr. John Winnie, Jesslyn Marie Braught, Lisa Hunter, and Cassandra Powell, as well as our illustrator Jessica Lohmeier, who were instrumental in capturing the visual aspect of the book.

In addition, books don't come to be without many other people, so we'd like to thank: all the people we've coached and worked with over the years, especially those who encouraged Melis to "write a book" or "shoot a video"—well...your wishes have come true; our "hydro" models/athletes (Ross Snider, Colter Mumford, Arianna Celis, Chris Edwards, Roger Fischer, Mitch Hanson, Trevon Hegel, and especially our cover runner/model, Bridget Hoopes) immortalized in press for all time; our lifeguards (Sam Garcia, Mary Buckingham, and Zoe Beardsley), keeping a safe eye during every underwater photo shoot; and finally our "readers," those people who read and re-read every word before going to press (Dr. Susan Burke, Mark and Rosie Fisher, Tom and Susan Snyder, Chris Edwards, Eric Wight, Kelly Fujikawa, Dr. John and Janet Winnie, Dr. Ryan and Suzie Clarke, Bridget Hoopes, and Tilda and Jerry Loftin). We deeply appreciate the encouragement and support we received from our friends and families during this process. Finally, we want to thank our spouses, Chris and Eric. They devotedly endured hours of us sitting and typing, inside, through wonderful Montana/Arizona summer days and spectacular evenings.

Thank you all,

Melis and Kat

From Kat: Melis, thank you for inviting me to join you in this adventure of a different kind, vastly expanding our horizons and our friendship. After 30 years, this is just the start.

From Melis: Kat, my friend, my sister in life. Thank you for making meaningful sentences out of what could've been considered written chaos.

About the Authors

In the fall of 1986, inside the anatomy lab at San Diego State University, Melis asked Kat to be her lab partner. Thus began a friendship that has spanned three decades and led to a collaboration that both say is the "best thing" they've ever done together. Author Melisenda Edwards and coauthor Katalin Wight exemplify the adage "opposites attract." Melis is flexible and impulsive while Kat is grounded and circumspect. But they each bring to the book their individual strengths and people skills.

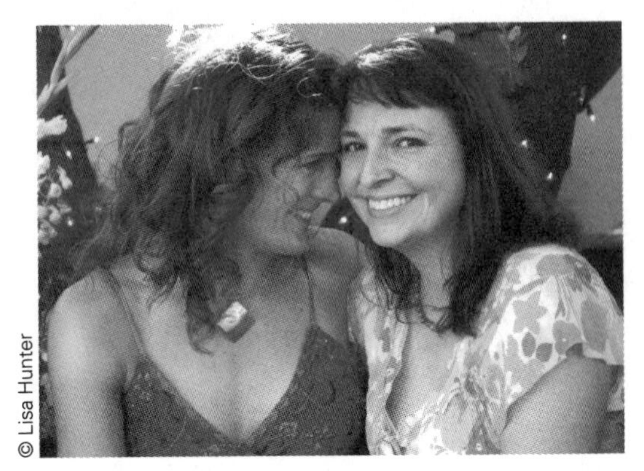

Melisenda Edwards (left) and Katalin Wight.

Over the last 30 years, **Melisenda "Mel" Edwards** has been a running and triathlon coach, personal trainer, fitness instructor, and, most importantly, athlete. Having participated in sports ranging from Ironman-distance triathlons to ultrarunning (including Western States 100), she understands the demands athleticism has on the body. With this knowledge, Melis has used the pool to work with athletes ranging from triathletes to professional hockey players, for training as well as rehabilitation. She holds a master's degree in health promotion and certifications with ACSM, as well as countless others. She lives in Belgrade, Montana.

An all-around athlete, **Katalin Wight** is an acute-care physical therapist with a master's degree in physical therapy from the University of California, San Francisco. Currently a runner and a hiker, she has been involved in organized sports since high school, participating in cross-country, rowing, track, hockey, and basketball. Kat brings a keen eye and experienced perspective to the techniques and methods that Melis has developed. She lives in Prescott, Arizona.

When together, Melis and Kat never run out of things to say, do, discuss, ponder, solve, and, of course, laugh about. They've taken countless trips together, even as far as New Zealand, talking and laughing no matter the mode of transportation—car, bus, plane, or on foot. As far as this book is concerned, these two friends have shared a dream and vision that align as smoothly as their work ethic. Their abilities blend seamlessly with one another, and their mutual respect and support of the other is unfailing. The authors have lived their lives in separate cities, yet they've experienced an uncanny parallelism—so it's not surprising that they're spreading their wings together with the culmination of this book.